I0434899

LOVE AFFAIR WITH MY HAIR

WHY BLACK WOMEN CHEAT ON HEALTH

HEATHER A. WORTHY & DR. DESIRÉE J. WILLIAMS

Always consult with your physician before you begin an exercise program or any type of physical activity. Never disregard medical advice or delay seeking it because of something you have read in **Love Affair with My Hair**. Any information in **Love Affair with My Hair** is meant for educational purposes and is not intended to be a substitute for any professional medical advice. All of the routines provided in this book should be performed at your own risk.

Copyright ©2014 Heather A. Worthy and Desirée J. Williams
All rights reserved.

ISBN-13: 978-1505575910
ISBN-10: 1505575915

CONTENTS

INTRODUCTION

The struggle between a black woman and her hair is real. In a world where first impressions are often determined based solely on appearance, the pressure to fit society's ideal image often veils the true essence of life: health and happiness. The amount of time and money we dedicate to our hair is exorbitant. Black women spend half a trillion dollars on hair care and weave products each year. Whether straight, wavy, curly, fine, or coarse, few things generate more passion among black women than their hair. But equally as difficult to fathom are the ever-growing health disparities between us and our Caucasian counterparts.

We have made vanity a top priority at the expense of our health. As a result of avoiding physical activity, obesity rates, along with the prevalence of stroke, heart disease, and diabetes are skyrocketing among black women. According to the U.S. Department of Health and Human Services, four out of five black women are overweight or obese, the highest rate in the country. While all of these health conditions have the potential to be fatal, they have also been scientifically proven to be largely preventable through maintaining a healthy diet and engaging in regular exercise. Nevertheless, we are held captive by the common phrase, "*I don't want to sweat my hair out!*"

The "*inconvenience*" of exercise is a real dilemma for black women and puts us in the position to have a love affair with our hair while we cheat on our health. Surgeon General Regina Benjamin explained that black women don't exercise due to the fact that it makes their hair go back to its natural state. Every black woman recognizes that water, whether it's from a pool, rain, sweat or the shower, is our worst enemy after a day at the hairdresser—a costly and time-consuming endeavor. The biggest challenge we face is retaining our hair style. Instead of changing the style we love, we can help each other and ourselves by finding creative solutions to this hold that our hair has over our health. This book will show you how to fine-tune your system so you can enjoy both good hair and great health.

Written for black women by two women who know your battle firsthand, this book is designed to educate, inspire, and lead you to a healthier lifestyle. We strive to motivate black women to become more fit; fit is not synonymous with thin, nor can every thin woman be considered fit. A fit woman integrates all of the components of health-related physical fitness along with a well-balanced diet into her daily routine. We will share styling and hair care tips, nutrition guidance and a comprehensive workout regimen. Pre-designed routines will allow you to schedule your exercise regimen around your visits to the hairdresser. We will also help you find a hairstyle that will work with physical activity. When all of this comes together, you will achieve success!

Equally important as the knowledge, we will provide a caring support system in order to motivate you on even your most tired days. That is why, along with the book, we have created an online community through which we support one another. Throughout the book, we encourage you to join us on our **Facebook** page (www.Facebook.com/LoveAffairWithMyHair), **Instagram** (LoveAffair_Hair), or **Twitter** (@LoveAffair_Hair), where we surround one another with positivity, support, motivation, and inspiration. None of us should feel alone on this journey; we are all here for one another! So let's put an end to the excuse of *"sweating out our hair"* once and for all.

We have built the body that we currently have by programming it to adapt to our habits and lifestyle. Joseph Pilates noted, *"Physical fitness can neither be achieved by wishful thinking nor outright purchase."* Simply put, thinking about working out burns exactly zero calories! It is important to keep in mind that everyone differs in their size, shape, appearance and fitness level so patience and perseverance are necessary when embarking on this journey to healthy living.

Just like taking a shower, brushing your teeth, eating or breathing, fitness should become a part of your everyday life. It is up to you to commit to a healthier lifestyle not only for yourself, but also for the health of your family and community for generations to come. You will make time for the things you deem important. So like your hair, make time to incorporate exercise into your everyday life. We are here to help you find real solutions to get you out of this love triangle between you, your hair and your health. So, if you're ready to have a healthy mind and body and a healthy head of hair, let's get started by taking this short survey! This is the first step to acknowledging and taking ownership of your personal habits and tendencies when it comes to your hair and exercise.

"Ability is what you're capable of doing. Motivation determines what you do. Attitude determines how well you do it."
American football player, coach, sportscaster, author, motivational speaker — Lou Holtz

TAKE THIS SHORT SURVEY!

1. How often do you schedule your hair appointment?
a. Less than once a month
b. Once a month
c. Twice a month
d. Once a week or more

2. How often do you wash and style your own hair?
a. 0-1 time/week
b. 2 times/week
c. 3 times/week
d. 4 or more times/week

3. On average, how much do you spend on your hair each month?
a. <$50
b. $50-100
c. $100-$150
d. >$150

4. I consider myself to be:
a. Fit and healthy
b. Healthy, but not fit
c. Mildly out of shape
d. Out of shape

5. How often do you participate in low to moderate exercise per week?
a. 0-1 time/week
b. 2 times/week
c. 3 times/week
d. 4 or more times/week

6. How often do you use your hair as an excuse not to exercise?
a. Never
b. Rarely
c. Sometimes
d. Always

7. Which one closely matches the reason as to why you don't exercise on a regular basis?
a. Time
b. Motivation
c. Hair
d. Other

CHAPTER 1

THE CULTURE OF HAIR AND THE BLACK WOMAN

Many black women take pride in the styling and presentation of their hair. Although we are often criticized for the value we place on the appearance of our manes, the importance of hair styling has been an integral part of black and African cultures for centuries. This means the maintenance of our hair extends far beyond its superficial context. In fact, the value of hair styling reaches back to our West African ancestry. Hair was used as a social indicator in West Africa; different hairstyles were used to represent marital status, age, religion, ethnicity, wealth, and even a person's surname.

Considering our history, it is clear why so many black women are obsessed with their hair. Black hair has always carried a level of societal influence and the significance of its styling has continued to transform throughout the centuries. As West Africans were transported to America to serve as slaves, many heads were shaved, symbolizing the destruction of West African culture and commencement of each slave's submission. As slaves' occupations were assigned, most slaves were forced to work long hours in the blistering sun, while few were appointed to domestic work in the master's home. Over time, enslaved women were forced to have affairs with their white masters resulting in offspring. These children not only had fairer skin, but also straightened, parted, or combed their hair to mimic their white owners'. In contrast, those slaves who worked outdoors were given little time nor resources to care for their hair. The result was matted, tangled hair often covered by scarves to protect it from the sun. This divide marked the beginning of black women's obsession with straight hair, as straight hair became viewed as more socially acceptable—closer to the white standard of beauty.

The desire for straight hair remained widespread until the Black Power movement exploded in the 1960s, encouraging black women to stop straightening their hair and instead embrace its natural state. The Black Power movement and its accompanying slogan "Black is Beautiful," are thought to be largely responsible for the popularity of the Afro. At that point in American history, one's hair began to represent one's political viewpoints.

As the Black Power movement concluded, African American culture again glorified straight, lustrous hair and shunned natural, kinky hair. The desire for hair that reflected European standards of beauty not only promoted the use of weaves, but also established a multi-billion dollar industry. Despite the economic recession and the expense associated with hair maintenance, hair salons remain among the most successful black businesses in urban communities.

After centuries of allowing our hair to possess more significance than owed, we finally moved into an era where black women have the option to choose any style they want. Many women rely on relaxers for more ease in styling, while others remain natural. Some women choose to wear dreads or braids, yet some choose flat irons and hair dryers. Black celebrities have helped broaden our nation's opinion of acceptable black hairstyles. Viola Davis proudly wore her TWA (teeny weeny afro) at the 2012 Academy Awards when nominated for Best Actress in a Leading Role. Singer Janelle Monae, landed the coveted Covergirl role while rocking her natural coif. As society has become more accepting of new ideas and opinions, black women now have greater freedom in choosing hairstyles without worrying about the political or social implications. However, regardless of hairstyle, the expectation is that hair must be kept neat and groomed in the professional workplace.

While most fitness experts would encourage changing hair to a more "workout-friendly" style, we should not—and do not—have to sacrifice our preferred style for our health. With that said, compromise is necessary. By the time you finish this book, you will have a solid foundation on how to create a balance between your health and your hair. Sporting great hair at the expense of your health is not worth forfeiting the improved quality of life that accompanies an active lifestyle. It is also important to consider the impact your lifestyle choices have on the people you value most.

We know each of you wears many hats; being a professional, a friend, a lover, a wife, a mother, and more, comes with much responsibility. Never underestimate the influence you have within each of your roles. Your lifestyle, in some way, affects your partner, spouse, coworkers, friends and especially your children. With the ever-growing obesity epidemic, it is time for you to become more conscious of the influence you have within your relationships. Habits, albeit good or bad, are contagious; a person is often a product of his or her surroundings. This manifestation is only augmented when raising children, who learn their most impactful life lessons through imitation. It is time to begin making a positive impression upon your family and community, and start on the path to better health.

Lastly, you are not the only woman trapped in this perpetual love triangle between you, your health, and your hair! You cannot continue to allow your hair to hold you and your health hostage. Together, with some preparation, we will be victorious. With any life-changing decision, you must first acknowledge your issues and roadblocks and make a commitment to change.

Start by visiting our **Facebook** page (**www.Facebook.com/LoveAffairWithMyHair**), **Instagram** (**LoveAffair_Hair**), or **Twitter** (**@LoveAffair_Hair**), to share your struggle. Use **#loveaffairwithmyhair** to tell us what your hair means to you. This is a great opportunity for you to interact and connect with other women who are confronting a similar conflict.

Now that you have confronted your problem, you can begin to resolve it by establishing a new target. Every year people make New Year's Resolutions. Unfortunately, research suggests that most people will never achieve those goals. Forbes magazine reports that while over 40% of Americans make New Year's Resolutions, less than 8% are successful in achieving them because their goals are not created with intention. In order to achieve a goal, it is important to follow a few guidelines:

Create a S.M.A.R.T. goal

Specific   Measurable   Attainable   Relevant   Time-bound

The best part is we have already done most of the work for you. This program encourages you to target improved health (specific and relevant) by committing to exercise at least three times a week (measurable) for a minimum of 12 weeks (time-bound). We have even outlined how to make this goal a reality (attainable) without sacrificing your hairstyle.

Write down your goal

Committing to your goal in writing not only helps you to visualize what you want, but also serves as a tool for reviewing your goals.

Establish a support system

It not enough to simply write down your goal; you must also proclaim your intentions to the people around you. You must share your goals with people who are willing and able to hold you accountable.

Review your progress

It is important to celebrate even the smallest victories throughout this process. That is why we have established weekly challenges, allowing you to acknowledge and share your successes over time.

We have provided you with a place to create, write, and review your goals. While you may have one overall goal, it is often difficult to stay motivated when your goal seems so far out of reach. For this reason, we have provided several goal sheets which outline how to develop several short-term goals en route to your final, long-term goal. Celebrate your small victories along the way; each time you make the choice to work out or select a healthy food option, you are one decision closer to the healthy woman you aspire to become.

Next, use **#hookupwithmyhealth** on Facebook, Twitter or Instagram to proclaim your goal. We challenge you to hookup with your health for at least 12 weeks while you complete this program. Once you make fitness a part of your routine, chances are you will want to continue this journey to improved health. In addition to your 12 week commitment, you may have other goals for yourself that you want to share with our online community. We welcome all positive commentary.

Be open. Be honest. But more importantly, be supportive of your sisters who share in your struggle. We are all striving for a common goal. Throughout this process, we can motivate and empower one another mentally, physically, and spiritually.

"Dream big, plan well, work hard, smile always, and good things will happen."
Artist and writer — Sally Huss

CHAPTER 2

BIG IS BEAUTIFUL, BUT AT WHAT COST?

While it is certainly possible to be big and beautiful, being overweight and healthy is much more difficult. Black America is long overdue for a "body-culture" revolution. For decades, black culture has praised voluptuous curves, thick thighs, and big hips, but have we gone too far? Too many women are tiptoeing along or have crossed the dangerous line between being "big-boned" (having a large frame) and being obese. Since four out of five black women are overweight or obese, we are 70% more likely to be obese than white women. It seems many black women are overweight by choice making it difficult to pinpoint the culprit for our high obesity rates.

Obesity-related diseases are killing our population at unparalleled rates. Nearly half of all blacks have been diagnosed with cardiovascular disease, making heart disease the leading cause of death for African Americans. In addition to heart disease, one in four middle-aged black women has diabetes—a diagnosis that is largely preventable through healthy eating and exercise. Due to the secondary diseases that accompany obesity, a direct correlation has been found between obesity and death in black women. The risk of death increases significantly as the Body Mass Index (BMI) rises above 25. Further, it should come as no surprise that these trends are trickling down to our children; more than one in four black girls is now considered obese.

Knowing these devastating statistics, why aren't black women running to the gym to combat this health issue? The answer may lie much deeper and it may be rooted in both politics and pop culture. Arguments have been made that a full-figured black woman serves as a refreshing juxtaposition to the image of the hard bodied slave. Dating back to the 18th Century, being slightly overweight was a sign of wealth and opulence among black and white populations. Fast-forward four centuries and decades-worth of research indicating the dangers of being overweight, and we now see a very distinct difference between the way white and black women view a plump body. According to a study by the Kaiser Family Foundation and *The Washington Post*, 66% of overweight black women had high self-esteem in comparison to only 41% of average-sized or thin white women. While it's wonderful that so many black women are comfortable in their own skin, without good health and longevity, confidence becomes secondary.

Through songs like Sir Mix-a-Lot's "Baby Got Back" and Soundmaster T's "2 Much Booty (In Da Pants)", black culture has applauded putting on extra weight. This ideal is compounded by the fact that we mask the description of being fat with more-desirable expressions like thick, healthy, or "big-boned". Others claim their desire to be full-figured is to combat the media's glorification of thinness. Regardless of whether it is a thin white woman or a full-figured black woman, both are adapting to a narrow aesthetic promoted by mainstream culture. It is time that we all end conformity, and stop making excuses to defend an unhealthy lifestyle. Instead of striving for a body type, we should strive for healthy hearts, strong muscles and bones, as well as the longevity that accompanies these characteristics.

Let's start by determining where you stand in the weight continuum. We will discuss two ways to determine your percentage of body fat. Although Body Mass Index calculations possess several inherent flaws, this measurement is relevant because much of the research surrounding obesity uses BMI as the criteria. BMI is calculated by a person's weight and height, and is used to determine a person's body fat percentage.

$$BMI = \frac{Weight\ (kg)}{Ht\ (m^2)} \qquad BMI = \frac{Weight\ (lbs)}{Ht\ (in^2)}$$

For example, a 5'5", 145-pound woman would have a BMI of 24.1.

Once you have determined your BMI, you can use that number to determine if your weight is within a healthy range:

Underweight: BMI is < 18.5   **Overweight:** BMI is 25-29.9
Normal Weight: BMI is 18.5-24.9   **Obese:** BMI is 30+

While we often use BMI as a standard for determining our body fat, it is important to note that BMI alone cannot gauge a person's level of health or fitness; it does not take body type or composition into consideration. BMI measurements do not distinguish between muscle mass and fat mass; therefore, it is possible to be underweight, yet still have poor fitness levels, and vice versa. However, BMI serves as a consistent guide in determining a person's healthy weight range, and is used to determine the statistics presented.

More recently, research has begun to promote a different gauge for percentage of body fat, called the Body Adiposity Index (BAI). Research on the BAI is still in its infancy and has not been tested among all ethnic groups. However, the BAI has been validated in African American and Mexican American populations. In contrast to BMI, BAI's formula uses a person's hip circumference and height. Keep in mind hip circumference is measured at the widest part of the hips around the buttocks.

$$BAI = \frac{\text{hip in cm}}{(\text{height in m})^{1.5}} - 18$$

Be mindful that the BAI equation uses metric measurements. That same 5'5'' woman would have to convert her height to 1.651 meters. Further, a woman with a hip circumference of 38 inches would have to convert her hip circumference to 96.52 centimeters. Using this equation, a 5'5'' woman with a hip circumference of 38 inches would have a BAI of 27.5%.

BAI ranges differ for men versus women. For the purpose of this text we have only included the ranges for women:

Age	Underweight	Healthy	Overweight	Obese
20-39	< 21%	21-33%	>33%	>39%
40-59	<23%	23-35%	>35%	>41%
60-79	<25%	25-38%	>38%	>43%

Once you know where you stand, you can use these values to track your progress to a healthier body. Though women have had to combat decades-worth of media brainwashing designed to condone black women being overweight, the feeling of being fit and healthy is unmatched. Not only will adopting a healthy lifestyle allow you to look your best, but you will also experience increased confidence, clarity of mind and sleep more soundly at night, to name a few benefits. In contrast to the lethal side effects of obesity, the results of making better food choices and being active are always positive. Now, let's get started on your journey to having fabulous hair and even better health!

"Make each day your masterpiece."
Basketball Hall of Famer and Basketball Coach — John Wooden

CHAPTER 3

STAYING FIT WITH A HEALTHY HEAD OF HAIR

"I don't want to sweat my hair out!"

We know that working out is good for us but it can be very hard on our hair. Black hair tends to be coarse so it dries out quickly, making skipping exercise after we get a fresh hairdo a common excuse among black women. Depending on our hairstyle, one visit to the gym can mess up our look, and it's challenging and time consuming to get presentable after leaving the gym. Many days, we choose maintaining our hair over working towards a healthier body. When we do this, we miss out on all of the health-boosting benefits of a workout.

While more common among women who regularly have their hair relaxed, women with all hairstyles and hair types have avoided exercise at one time or another. Women's concerns about "sweating out their hair" are due to the amount of time it takes to wash, dry, and style hair, or may be attributed to the itchy scalp many experience once sweat dries. The exercise program in this book schedules more strenuous exercise immediately prior to your already scheduled hair-washing.

In this chapter, we will offer hair care solutions to show you how healthy hair can be maintained and your hairstyle preserved during and after exercise. You will be surprised to learn how easy it is to care for your hair when you adopt a simple pre and post-workout hair care regimen. Whether you are at home or in the locker room, you can use these tips to make your hair look great, allowing you to say goodbye to rough hair days and wasted gym membership fees.

To maintain the integrity of hair while working out, the most important thing to remember is to keep your hair moisturized. When the natural salt in our sweat combines with our hair, it often dehydrates the hair shaft, leaving hair brittle and more susceptible to breakage. Immediately following a workout, it is crucial to replenish our hair's moisture using a product specifically designed for its thickness.

For those individuals who have a finer grade of hair—or those who feel their scalp becomes oily quickly—light, thin oil should be used. Common light hair oils include pure argan oil, coconut oil, grape seed oil, and jojoba oil. These oils are usually transparent and do not leave a greasy feel. On the other hand, those individuals who have thicker or coarser hair may require denser oil like olive oil or castor oil in order to provide hair with lasting moisture.

When determining the right oil for your hair type, sometimes the best answer is found by trial and error. Remember, regardless of how you style your hair—relaxed, natural or weave—it is important to keep your hair moisturized.

Caring for Relaxed Hair

Even though relaxed hair undergoes controlled damage, maintaining the health of chemically straightened hair is possible. All hair should be pampered, but relaxed hair requires special treatment due to its processed nature. These seven tips for maintaining healthy relaxed hair can help you get your straight tresses into great shape. All you need are the right tools, products and a little patience!

Relax your hair every 8 to 12 weeks depending on your hair's needs. Relaxing your hair every time new growth appears can cause damage to the hair. For one week following your relaxer, use a reconstructor instead of your regular conditioner when you wash your hair.

Wash and condition your hair once or twice a week. Try to use mild and gentle shampoo and conditioner designed for chemically treated hair. Using a deep conditioner that contains both protein and moisture once per week is ideal in conjunction with some type of heat element to open up the hair cuticle. A hair steamer or a hot wet towel wrapped around the head with a shower cap both work well. Regular and consistent deep conditioning can help maintain the hair's integrity, allowing it to withstand regular manipulation and styling.

Chemically treated hair must always be treated with a leave-in conditioner after every wash. Wet hair is in its most vulnerable state and is more likely to break than dry hair. Combing the wet hair with a wide tooth comb or shower/detangling comb will prevent breakage. For those who need to wash more frequently than once or twice a week, conditioner-only washing (also known as co-washing) is an excellent alternative to the typical wash/condition. For best results, simply rinse the hair well with warm water, apply conditioner to the hair starting 1-2 inches away from the scalp, smooth it through to the ends, and rinse well.

It is best to avoid using heat to dry your hair, especially if the relaxed hair is somewhat damaged. Hair should be left to air dry at least partially before using a blow dryer on a low to medium temperature setting. However, if your hair is healthy and you prefer heat, you can either blow dry on medium or use a hood dryer with magnetic rollers. The hair should be completely dry before you use a curling or flat iron on it. Flat irons and curling irons are very convenient, but daily use will eventually lead to dryness and damage. Make sure to use a heat protection product prior to any heat use.

An ionic, ceramic curling iron or flat iron works well and is easy to find. You should also invest in quality heat appliances that have temperature controls. Relaxed hair can easily be styled at 300-370 degrees depending on the hair's thickness. Do not repeatedly run the heat appliance over each section of hair. Instead, pass the iron over the hair once or twice at this temperature. A great technique for ensuring your hair gets straight with a single pass is to section your hair then use a fine toothed comb to hold the hair taut, leaving just enough room to fit the flat iron in between the comb and your scalp. Use the fine toothed comb to guide the flat iron to the end of the strand. Again, it's important to use heat protective products, but not oils, prior to all heat styling.

Keeping the hair and scalp moisturized. Depending on your hair type, you may need to use hair moisturizer daily. For best results, choose a lightweight oil (such as jojoba, coconut, almond, or olive oil). To use the oil on dry hair, rub a small amount (1-2 drops) in the palms of your hands, and spread lightly through the scalp. Next, comb your hair evenly to moisturize the tips of the hair.

Wrap and Protect at Night. Not only does wrapping your hair at night save you styling time in the morning, but it also protects your hair while you sleep. Molding your hair to the shape of your head is a low-maintenance way to protect your hair from excessive heat while preserving its body and volume. Using extra protection like a silky hair cover or pillowcase will help as well.

Caring for a Relaxed Short Style versus a Relaxed Mid-Length or Longer

Whether you have short hair or mid-length to longer hair, additional work is required immediately before and after a workout. Before working out, if you have short hair use a dime-sized amount of oil to lay the hair down. If you have mid-length to longer styles use a quarter sized to do the same. Prior to working out, a dime to quarter-sized amount of oil should be used to lay the hair down. These precautions will keep your hair moisturized while you sweat.

If you have mid-length to longer hair, you can wear your hair in a ponytail while working out. Using a roller or two at the end of the hair prevents breakage. It will also help keep your hair off your neck without causing unnecessary bends that often accompany wearing your hair in a bun or braid. Additionally when the tip of your ponytail brushes against the sweat on your neck, even that small contact with sweat can cause your ends to dry out. Remember, protecting your ends are important to maintaining an overall healthy head of hair.

After the workout, remove the headband. If you did not sweat enough to alter the appearance of your hair, wear it that way. If your hair has become damp during the workout, use a heat-protective serum or light oil prior to using the blow dryer and flat iron. Make sure that the roots are dry by using the blow dryer on a low temperature setting prior to using the flat iron on a low setting (300 degrees) to straighten or "bump curl" the hair.

For longer hair, you can wear your hair back in a single bun or buy hair in the form of a bun and bring your hair into it. Adding a single braid or twist around the edges of the hair is also a stylish way to camouflage your edges without applying additional heat. Just remember that wet hair is in a fragile state, so allow your edges to dry before attempting to manipulate it into a braid or twist, and add oil to maintain moisture. On the other hand, short hairstyles are a great option for physically active black women, and can be washed and styled more frequently without breakage being an issue. With this hairstyle, the physically active black woman can create a sophisticated look in minutes.

Caring for Natural Hairstyles

Due to its naturally coiled shape, black hair tends to be dry and requires less-frequent washing than other hair types. However, when exposed to sweat, the hair needs to be washed more regularly to avoid the buildup of impurities and to keep it from becoming too dry. One option for those who do not want to expose their hair to heat damage from frequent flat ironing is to consider a natural hairstyle. Although some natural styles require extensive styling after washing, there is also the option of wearing a wash-and-go style, an Afro, a bun, or a curly ponytail.

Here are some general tips to ensure you are taking good care of your natural tresses:

Wash and condition your hair 2-3 times a week using the right products. Many women are frightened about washing too much, but the proper products will actually restore the moisture to your natural tresses. Use mild shampoos, and avoid shampoo products that contain sodium laureth sulfate or alcohol. There are several products on the market labeled sulfate-free. Sulfate is a traditional shampoo ingredient which can strip the hair of its natural moisture. You will likely have to scan the list of ingredients in your hair products to confirm the product does not contain alcohol.

Like relaxed hair, natural hair also benefits from using a deep conditioner that contains both protein and moisture once per week. This deep conditioner should be used with some type of heat element to open up the hair cuticles. Deep conditioning regularly and consistently can help maintain the hair's integrity, allowing it to withstand regular manipulation and styling, as well as preventing damage. If you are one of those individuals who prefer daily hair washing, conditioner-only washing is an excellent option for you. Simply rinse your hair with warm water and apply conditioner 1-2 inches away from the scalp. Apply conditioner to the hair and smooth it through to the ends, applying more to the ends if they are dry. Then, thoroughly rinse the conditioner from your hair.

Blot-dry hair with a towel. Instead of squeezing or wringing out the hair after washing, blot hair with a towel to preserve the hair's curl pattern.

Comb hair using your fingers. Instead of using a comb that can disrupt the natural curl pattern of your hair, use your fingers as a comb.

Keep hair sufficiently moisturized. Since black hair is naturally dry, you need products that are extremely moisturizing. Moisturize hair daily using water-based moisturizers or coconut oil, and avoid products with petroleum, lanolin, sodium laureth sulfate and alcohol.

Caring for Natural Hair Worn Straight

There are many black women who have natural, non-chemically treated hair, but choose to wear their hair in a heat-straightened style. For those women, we recommend you follow the same protocol as for women with relaxed hair.

Caring for Natural Hair in a Short Style

Short, natural hair is one of the best options for the active black woman. Although it's important to remember to keep hair moisturized, short hair requires little to no styling before and after a workout; most short styles can be styled by adding a moisturizing product or by using a wash-and-go method.

Caring for Natural Hair that is Mid-Length or Longer

Before you workout, put your hair into big twists or divide hair into four braids. Since sweat will dry out your hair, you should also wear a scarf or a headband to wick away your sweat so the hair absorbs less moisture. After your workout, you can simply unravel hair for a wavy look, adding more water or product if necessary. It may be helpful to keep a spray bottle with water to add moisture without having to submerge your hair in water. Another option is to wash or wash/condition your hair and wear it in a wash-and-go style.

Wearing a Protective Style

As more black women begin to adopt active lifestyles, protective styles are becoming increasingly common. Common protective styles include braids, twists, wraps, buns, and full-headed weaves, to name a few. If you are finding difficulty with doing your hair after working out, you may want to try one.

When deciding on a protective style, it's important to work with a stylist that is careful to maintain the health and integrity of your hair. Some stylists may pull hair too tightly and braid or twist it too small, resulting in more of the breakage you were trying to avoid.

Additionally, protective styles cannot be kept in too long or your hair will begin to tangle and lock. It's important to continue to care for you hair, even in its protective style. You must regularly rinse hair after excessive sweating and keep hair moisturized using oil. Regardless of the way in which you choose to style and wear your hair, maintaining the integrity of your hair is important; don't be afraid to give your hair a little TLC.

"A healthy attitude is contagious but don't wait to catch it from others. Be a carrier".
— Tom Stoppard, British Playwright and Screenwriter

CHAPTER 4

YOU ARE WHAT YOU EAT: HEALTHY IS THE NEW BEAUTIFUL

The statistics on the prevalence of overweight and obese Americans are depressing. To many black women, a big body is beautiful and represents health and prosperity, but does being thin or big really represent being beautiful? The black female is in crisis when it comes to our health and one of the main culprits is our diet. Yes, black culture and heredity may play a role, but we need to be honest with ourselves and understand that some of this obesity crisis is self-inflicted. We don't exercise like we should for a variety of reasons (socioeconomic, demographic and psychosocial) and we often choose to ignore or remain uneducated regarding how the food industry manufactures what we consume daily. The quantity and quality of our diets have evolved such that we can eat unhealthy foods virtually non-stop.

According to the CDC (Centers for Disease Control), 80% of black women are either overweight or obese. Obesity is linked to our developing heart disease, diabetes, cancer and high cholesterol at double the rates of our non-black counterparts. Black women must be willing to discuss the real issue of obesity if we are to address the health disparities that make us and our families live unhealthy and shorter lives.

While it is okay to encourage personal behaviors like healthy eating and physical activity as a part of the solution to the problem, we must also address the structural factors that undermine our health. To do so, we need to support each other and collaborate with schools, religious and community groups, businesses, and government leaders to reshape our communities into places where healthier choices are made readily accessible. Regardless of whether you're rich or poor, old or young, single parenting or married, in the daily grind of working in the corporate world, or a small-business owner, you're likely experiencing some level of stress that is affecting your health on a daily basis. We all struggle to maintain good health in this modern world of convenience. No one said it would be easy, but we will come together to tackle this obesity crisis one step at a time.

The spirit of black culture has been passed down by storytelling through generations in the African tradition and through the preparation of "soul" food. A black woman's illustration of love, character, cultivation, originality, stamina, defeat, resilience, and her African legacy are at the heart of her meal planning. Soul food is also considered "comfort" food because it makes us feel happy, safe and tastes so good! But besides the extra serving of love that gets put into making soul food, what makes it taste so good? The answer is sugar, fat and salt.

Sugar, fat and salt—principal ingredients in all of the foods that we love—are at the forefront of the obesity epidemic in America. These foods, which we know are not good for us, make up about 61% of our diets. America's food industry has transitioned from a nation of enjoying farm fresh food to one that mass-produces and pre-packages most of what we eat. This preparation adversely affects the quality of what we consume. The typical American diet exceeds the recommended intake levels or limits in four categories: calories from solid fats and added sugars; refined grains; sodium; and saturated fat. Americans eat less than the recommended amounts of vegetables, fruits, whole-grains, dairy products, and oils and eat more sodium than is recommended for a healthy diet. For this reason, scaling back on our portion sizes is secondary to the questioning of what it is that we are putting into our bodies. Food has effects on the body that can either be devastating or life saving. It has been proven that many chronic illnesses can be avoided by simply cooking and eating healthy foods. As black women, we need to be more aware of what we consume and prepare for our families.

These days, we have a wealth of nutritional information at our fingertips and everyone seems to have an opinion about what you should and shouldn't eat. You may find it difficult to decipher all of this information about nutrition and food choices. Nevertheless, it's no secret that good nutrition plays an essential role in maintaining health. Let's start by discussing some basic nutrition information.

The five food groups consist of vegetables, fruits, grains, dairy and proteins. The vegetables and fruits you eat may be fresh, frozen, canned or dried and may be eaten whole, cut-up, mashed or pureed. When selecting frozen or canned fruits, be sure to choose options without added sugar; fruits contain natural sugars, so adding additional sugar will quickly turn a healthy fruit into a sugar-filled dessert.

You should also eat a variety of dark green, red and orange vegetables. Similar to fruits, vegetables also come in many forms. When eating canned vegetables choose the low-sodium option. Many frozen vegetables are flash-frozen, therefore maintaining their nutrient levels. In some instances, frozen vegetables actually contain higher nutrient values. However, make sure to avoid the frozen vegetables topped with butter or cheese.

There are two types of grains: whole grains and refined grains. At least half of the grains you eat should be whole grains. Whole grains provide a variety of health benefits which includes a reduction in the risk of heart disease and other chronic diseases, weight management, proper bowel function, and the fostering of a healthy immune system. Additionally, they are great for our waistlines. Examples of whole grains include oatmeal, whole wheat and rye, brown and wild rice, and whole grain cereals.

All milks and calcium-containing milk products, such as cheese and yogurt, count in the dairy category.   However, most of your dairy choices should be fat-free or low-fat milk products. Still, many low-fat dairy-based snacks, particularly yogurt, are often loaded with sugar; always check the nutrition label to ensure your dairy snacks aren't full of sugar.

Lastly, in the protein group, choose a variety of lean meats and poultry, seafood, beans and peas, eggs, processed soy products, unsalted nuts, and seeds. Lean proteins have 50-60 calories and 2-3 grams of fat per serving. One ounce is considered a serving. A serving is a measured amount of food or drink. A portion is the amount of food you choose to eat. Portions tend to be larger than one serving for the protein group. Four to six ounces is the suggested amount for lean proteins. These include foods such as the white meat of chicken or turkey with the skin removed, salmon, lean beef that has "round", "chuck", or "loin" in its name, low-fat cheese and pork tenderloin.

These five groups are the building blocks for a healthy diet, but more and more we see that Americans are falling short when it comes to their diet and eating clean and healthy foods.

Eating clean is a good way to refresh your eating habits and does not focus on counting calories. Instead, it emphasizes eating more of the best and healthiest options in each of the food groups and eating less of the not-so-healthy ones. Eating clean means limiting processed, packaged foods and increasing whole, fresh foods like vegetables, fruits, whole grains, healthy proteins, and fats. It also means cutting back on refined grains, added sugars, salt, and unhealthy saturated fats.

Here are some tips regarding eating a well-balanced and clean diet. We are sure you will find these tips to be helpful and a great starting point!

Balance Calories - Find out how many calories you need for a day to help you manage your weight. This depends on your age, height, weight, gender, daily activity level, metabolic rate and if you want to lose, gain or maintain your weight. One method to find your estimated daily caloric maintenance level is to take your current weight and multiply it by 14 and then by 17 to get your range. For example, a 150lb person would calculate 150 x 14 and 150 x 17 and get an estimated daily calorie maintenance level of somewhere between 2100-2550 calories. Various smart phone applications are available to calculate this information as well.

Enjoy Your Food - Stop and consider whether you are really hungry or just bored. If you determine that you are actually hungry, keep your portions reasonable, take the time to fully enjoy your food and avoid eating quickly.

Avoid Oversized Portions - Use a smaller plate, bowl or glass. Portion out foods before you eat. When eating out, choose a smaller sized serving, share a dish, or take home part of your meal. Remember to wait at least twenty minutes before you go up for "seconds". This time period allows for some digestion to take place. If you just wait, you will probably feel full and satisfied. Try it and see!

Eat Good Foods More Often - Think about what you can add to your diet, not what you can take away. Eat more vegetables, fruits, whole grains, and fat-free milk and dairy products.

Fruits and Vegetables - Focus on adding the recommended 5-9 servings of fruit and vegetables each day. Work vegetables into meals instead of just serving them as side dishes.

Switch to Fat-Free or Low-Fat (1%) Milk - These products have the same amount of calcium and other essential nutrients as whole milk, but fewer calories and less saturated fat.

Make Half Your Grains Whole Grains - Substitute a whole-grain product for a refined product such as brown rice for white rice. Avoid foods made with doughy and buttery breads, biscuits and croissants.

Foods to Eat Less Often - Cut back on foods high in solid fat, added sugar and salt like cakes, sweetened drinks and pizza. Use these foods as occasional treats, not every day foods.

Compare Sodium in Foods - The Nutrition Facts label is your friend. Select foods labeled "low sodium", "reduced sodium", or "no salt added".

Drink Water instead of Sugary Beverages - Cut calories by drinking plenty of water and other unsweetened calorie-free beverages. Try not to confuse thirst with hunger. Drinking a glass of water when you feel hungry will help to alleviate the hunger pains and will oftentimes lead to decreased food consumption.

Keep in mind that the key to weight control is balancing your food intake and your physical activity. The recommended amount of calories a person needs per day is highly specific to each individual depending on gender, age, height, and level of daily activity. However, the benchmark number, as seen on food labels, is approximately 2,000 calories per day. Having said that, when you consume only as many calories as your body needs, your weight will usually remain constant. Consequently, if you take in more calories than your body needs, you will put on excess weight. In order to burn excess fat you must expend more energy than you take in. Therefore, exercise plays an important role in weight control by increasing energy output and using stored calories for extra fuel.

Exercise raises your metabolism during a workout and your metabolism remains elevated for an extended period of time after exercising, allowing you to burn more calories. The concept of metabolism remaining elevated following a workout explains why so many fitness professionals encourage morning workouts. Increasing your heart rate--and therefore metabolism--early in the morning could potentially help you burn more calories all day long.

The other component of meal planning is meal preparation. We are all busy and it is easy to be tempted by fast food; therefore, if you can spend some time each Sunday packing lunches and preparing the ingredients for your weekday meals, you will be much more inclined to make good food choices and stay compliant with your meal planning.

Furthermore, we would be remiss if we didn't briefly discuss the effects of overeating as well as under-eating, as both can have negative effects on our health. People overeat due to boredom, depression, or as the result of bad habits. There are many reasons one should be stopped before the habit gets out of control. Overeating may cause weight gain, nutrient deficiencies, diabetes, heart disease, hypertension, depression, chronic fatigue, irregular menses, nausea, kidney disease, arthritis, bone deterioration, and stroke. Conversely, under-eating is done for various reasons including losing weight, depression, or simply because of a busy lifestyle. Some of the results of under-eating include malnutrition, reproductive problems, low bone density, hypoglycemia, wasted body tissue, suppressed immune function, low blood pressure, hair loss, gallstones, weakness, and lack of energy. The best way to break these bad habits is to eat scheduled meals and snacks. Meal planning isn't always easy, but when you stick with it you will find that it works.

So what about fast food? Should we never eat at a fast food restaurant? While we aren't advocates of fast food, we wouldn't go as far as to say never because for some, fast food may be the only option. For many others, busy schedules force us to occasionally visit a drive-thru. If you do end up at the drive–thru window, you have the power to choose healthier menu options. Avoid fried foods, choose smaller portions like a small fry instead of the large version, and be aware of the sugary, high calorie beverages you pair with a meal. Did you know that a 20-ounce bottle of soda contains the equivalent of approximately 16 teaspoons of sugar? The American Heart Association recommends we consume no more than five to nine teaspoons per day. If you order a salad, choose a vinegar-based dressing as opposed to a cream-based dressing like ranch; to reduce refined carb intake, remove half of the hamburger bun. These quick tips give you many more options if you find yourself in a predicament of choosing fast food or starving.

Another small tip is to order items on the value menu; these are smaller servings than the outrageous portions elsewhere on the menu. The result will be a meal with fewer calories and fat grams. Most fast food companies offer healthier options and display a calorie guide for each menu item. Take advantage and use this information to help you make better decisions. Remember, fast food chains are not the only culprit in this obesity crisis. There are many other casual and fine dining restaurants that have unhealthy options on their menu as well. Anytime you dine out, you have to be careful with your food selections and make better decisions in order to live a healthier lifestyle when it comes to your diet.

Ladies, we can't eat perfectly all the time. It is impossible and will likely cause unnecessary stress if we attempt to do so. However, we can try to be more conscious of what we do consume regardless of whether we are preparing it, dining out or eating fast food. Keep in mind that we all deserve a "cheat" meal to enjoy the foods we love, but should do so in moderation and after we have earned it through increased physical activity. Remember that if we consume more calories than we expend, we will gain weight, and gaining weight could be counterproductive to our goal of living a longer and healthier life. Healthy is the new beautiful. Let's help each other get there together!

"Where there is no struggle, there is no strength."
Media proprietor, talk show host, actress,
producer, philanthropist — Oprah Winfrey

CHAPTER 5

KEEPING AN ACTIVE EXERCISE ROUTINE IN THIRTY MINUTES OR LESS

"No…I don't want to sweat my hair out!" It's like we are stuck in this repetitive cycle and are helpless due to our obsession. We feel forced to choose between working out and having great hair. The reality is that we can have both.

We previously shared some of the hair challenges that we encounter when we sweat. Our hair tends to feel dry, look frizzy, and lack luster while our scalp annoyingly itches. Even when we work out with a scarf, pins or a mesh cap on our heads desperately trying to preserve our hair, it is never easy to get our hair back to the look we desire. It is often viewed as too hard and time consuming to look presentable after exercise, but we must find a way to get over that hump.

Getting fit is more than before and after pictures. It's more than what the scale reads or what our hair looks like. Being fit is about feeling healthy on the inside and outside and creating a body built to last. We know that exercise helps us look and feel better; now, we just have to put our knowledge into practice. Remember, we can enjoy our workouts and have great hair too. This journey is not a sprint; instead, it's a marathon, and we are so happy you will let us guide you to the finish line!

Before you begin any exercise program, knowing your medical history is important. If you have any condition such as high blood pressure, diabetes, cardiac issues or any other "red flags", these may require medical clearance from your physician. It is necessary to have a comprehensive understanding of some key pieces of information, including your physical readiness for activity, general lifestyle information and medical history. Remember, fitness is influenced by age, gender, heredity, personal habits, exercise, and eating practices. The first three factors can't be changed which is why it is imperative to know your medical history, but the latter three can be improved when you make the commitment to do so.

A well-designed fitness-training program includes a healthy diet, increased water intake, exercise and rest. These lifestyle habits encourage your body to continually move in a fit and healthy direction. The body functions best when it is active regularly and receives the necessary nutrients to support this function. All of the systems that make up your body support each other and function in harmony when your body is busy adapting to maximize its healthy potential.

Carrying out a fitness program takes time, effort and patience. Achieving healthy living is a lifelong process for everyone. Your goals will constantly evolve and there will be successes and challenges along the way. If you work hard and stay committed you can achieve the healthy lifestyle that you have always wanted. Here are some tips to ensure your workouts are successful.

View Exercise as Fun - Exercise should be fun! By choosing activities that are appealing or interesting, you combine the benefits of fitness with enjoyment. People who view exercise as an undesirable chore have a hard time doing it and will find it much harder to attain their goals.

Set Realistic Goals - Set appropriate and measurable goals that start from where you are and progress at a reasonable rate. Unrealistic or vague goals can contribute to exercise dropout. Remember, you can't regain in a few days or weeks what you have lost in months or years of sedentary living. Try to define challenging but not impossible goals. Typically, weight loss at a rate of 1-2 lbs/week is a healthy rate at which to lose weight. "Strive for progress, not perfection."-Unknown

Exercise with a Purpose and Take a Day Off - Exercise with a purpose and improve the quality of each movement. Your workouts will take half of the time when you push yourself to perform at optimal capacity. Our workouts are designed to take thirty minutes or less, three days out of the week with four rest days in between! Taking a day or two off between workouts is just as important as the physical activity and you will see better results when you do.

Track Your Exercise and Eating Habits - Keep an exercise log and food journal to track your exercise and break the cycle of poor eating habits.

Do the Right Type of Workout for Your Body - The exercise you are doing directly determines your results. Make sure you are doing the right type of workout designed to meet your goals.

Understand How the Body Works - You cannot spot reduce. To reduce fat in a particular area of the body, you need an overall reduction of body fat, which is achieved from a healthy diet, regular and consistent exercise and proper rest. If your diet is poor and you don't engage in regular cardiovascular activity such as biking, walking, running or kickboxing, you can do 1,000 sit ups a day and never have a "flat stomach".

Change Your Workout - Doing the same workout over and over can lead to burnout as well as boredom. Avoid hitting a plateau and change your workouts every 4 to 6 weeks.

Measure the Right Results - Don't rely solely on what the scale says. Ask yourself how you feel mentally and physically. Compare where you were when you started your fitness journey to where you are now. Maybe you can perform more burpees or push ups after a month of working out than you could before. Check out the fitness challenge exercises (pg. 69, pg. 85, pg. 101) and track your progress.

Use Correct Form and Technique - Form matters when you exercise. Incorrect form and technique can lead to injuries, pain and soreness. We have added pictures and cues in this chapter to make sure you are performing the exercises properly and maximizing your workouts.

"Good" Pain versus "Bad" Pain - Knowing the difference between pain and muscle soreness during or after exercise is important. There is a definite distinction between the two and it is important to recognize each. Pain is your body's way of telling you that you are doing too much or performing a move incorrectly; this is the "bad" pain. A sharp or jabbing sensation is a signal for injury and means you should take it easy and seek medical advice if the pain persists. In contrast, muscle soreness is a signal that you're doing more than you are used to doing. This is typical when you begin any new workout program; this is the "good" pain. Good pain is generally felt three to four hours after exercise and can be felt as much as two to three days later. You can still exercise with this type of pain and the soreness will eventually subside.

Next, we will discuss a very simple exercise principle, F.I.T.T., and what each of these initials means. This will help you understand the 12 week workout regimen we have created for you. **Frequency (F)** is the number of times per week that you will train. **Intensity (I)** is how hard you train. **Time (T)** is the duration of each training session and **Type (T)** is the type of exercise being performed. Our program allows you to workout at three different intensity levels throughout the week: light, moderate and hard. We have outlined a workout regimen with a frequency of three times a week, planned around your hair appointment schedule. The initial workouts utilize only your body weight. As the weeks progress, the exercises become more challenging and you will have the option of adding light to moderate resistance using dumbbells and/or tubing. On the light days, your hair should virtually feel and look untouched. On the moderate days, you can expect to sweat some. On the hard days, plan on "sweating your hair out".

Although we have given you an exercise plan for three days per week, we encourage you to add a fourth or fifth day incorporating aerobic activities such as walking, jogging, taking the stairs, biking, or even dancing. While strength training requires rest days, it is safe to do cardiovascular exercise on a daily basis. Remember, choose activities that you enjoy and make exercise fun!

Your exercise schedule is based solely on what works best for you. It is important to schedule your workouts for a time when there is little chance that you will have to cancel or interrupt them because of other demands on your time or your hair. The bottom line is you will make time for the things that you want to do in your life. Make exercise your new friend and leave the excuses at the door. Charles Buxton said, "You will never find time for anything. If you want time, you must make it."

Now on to the fun part of getting you out of this love triangle between you, your health and your hair! We have already given you hair care tips and different hairstyle options, in addition to nutrition and fitness tips. It's time to put all of that knowledge together and make a plan! The following charts were created to help you stay on track with your exercise program and your hair appointments or hair-washing days. Typically, hair salons are open Tuesday through Saturday (if you happen to get your hair done on a Sunday or Monday, you can adjust the schedule). However, we encourage you to keep a similar format regarding your light (L), moderate (M), hard (H) and off days. We have made short and easy-to-follow routines with pictures and cues for the next twelve weeks. Keep in mind that your regimen will change every four weeks to keep your body guessing and improve your results. Make sure to journal and complete your goal sheets. It has been proven that those who journal hold themselves accountable and are two to three times more likely to see results.

Don't forget about our online community. Join us on our **Facebook** page (**www. Facebook.com/LoveAffairWithMyHair**), **Instagram** (**LoveAffair_Hair**), and **Twitter** (**@ LoveAffair_Hair**) to get support, motivation, inspiration, and tell us and others about how you are doing with the program. Let's have fun, achieve a healthy lifestyle, and make sure we stay committed to never cheating on our health again!

*"If you don't like something, change it.
If you can't change it, change your attitude."*
Author, poet, dancer, actress and singer — Maya Angelou

12 WEEK WORKOUT REGIMEN BASED ON YOUR HAIR APPOINTMENT SCHEDULE

SELECT THE CALENDAR BELOW THAT HIGHLIGHTS YOUR "HAIR-WASHING DAY" AND FOLLOW THAT SCHEDULE

H Hard Routine (High Intensity) Heavy Sweat Day
M Moderate Routine (Moderate Intensity) Moderate Sweat Day
L Light Routine (Low Intensity) Mild to No Sweat Day

TUESDAY APPOINTMENT

MONDAY	TUESDAY	WEDNESDAY	THURSDAY	FRIDAY	SATURDAY	SUNDAY
H	Hair Apt.	Off	L	Off	M	Off

WEDNESDAY APPOINTMENT

MONDAY	TUESDAY	WEDNESDAY	THURSDAY	FRIDAY	SATURDAY	SUNDAY
Off	H	Hair Apt.	Off	L	Off	M

THURSDAY APPOINTMENT

MONDAY	TUESDAY	WEDNESDAY	THURSDAY	FRIDAY	SATURDAY	SUNDAY
M	Off	H	Hair Apt.	Off	L	Off

FRIDAY APPOINTMENT

MONDAY	TUESDAY	WEDNESDAY	THURSDAY	FRIDAY	SATURDAY	SUNDAY
Off	M	Off	H	Hair Apt.	Off	L

SATURDAY APPOINTMENT

MONDAY	TUESDAY	WEDNESDAY	THURSDAY	FRIDAY	SATURDAY	SUNDAY
L	Off	M	Off	H	Hair Apt.	Off

YOU ARE BEGINNING WEEK 1

Starting Weight _____   Date _____

- Short-Term Goals:

_____

_____

_____

- Intermediate Goals:

_____

_____

_____

- Long-Term Goals:

_____

_____

_____

- Ultimate Goals:

_____

_____

_____

- I plan to reach my goal by:

- I will do the following to reach my goal:

- I can imagine myself:

- I will track my progress by:

- Potential personal and fitness challenges that I may face in the next 4 weeks are:

- My reward for reaching my goal will be:

- I believe and expect that I can:

WEEKS 1 THROUGH 4 ONLY

LIGHT DAY: 20 MINUTE WORKOUT

5 x 10 x 5 ROUTINE
(5 Exercises x 10 Repetitions x 5 Sets)
Squat
Pushup
Side Lunge (10 each leg)
Russian Twist (10 each side)
Jumping Jack
***Perform the five exercises in the set with the given amount of repetitions.
Rest thirty seconds to one minute then repeat until the five sets are completed.***

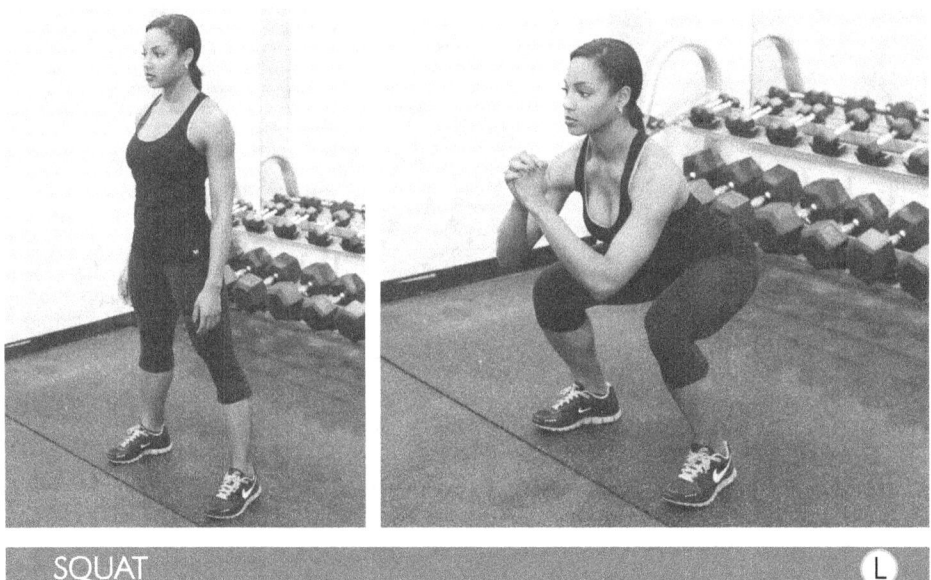

SQUAT

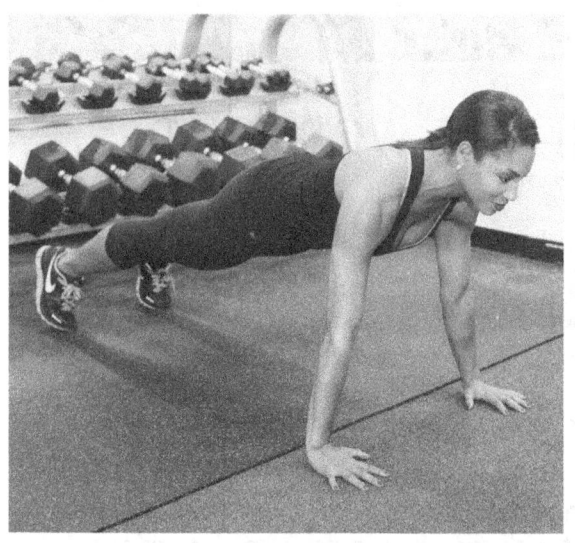
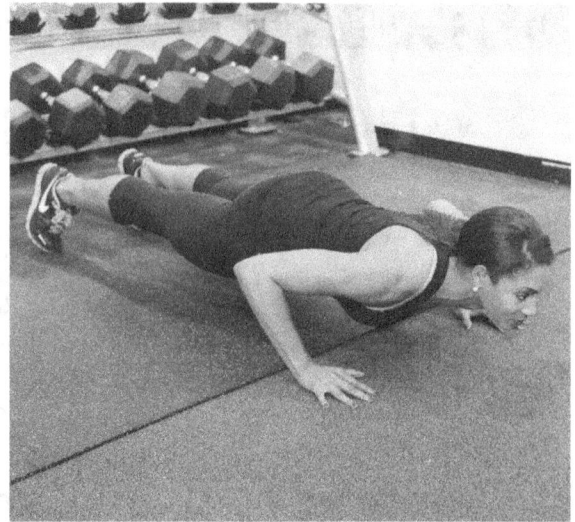

PUSH-UP   Ⓛ

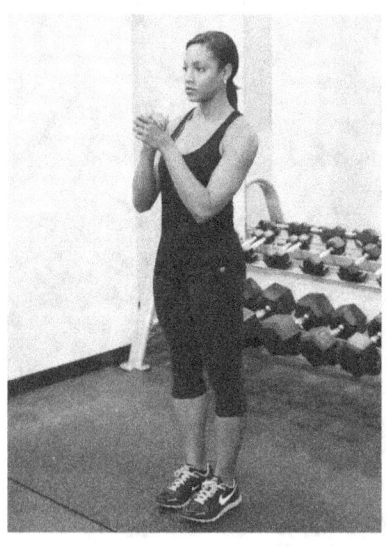
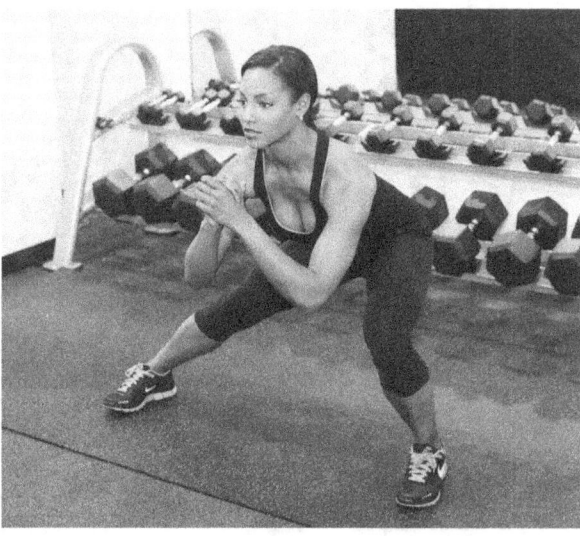

SIDE LUNGE   Ⓛ

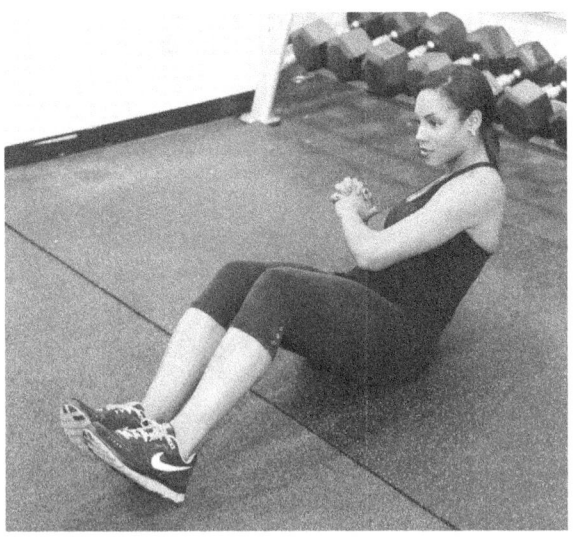
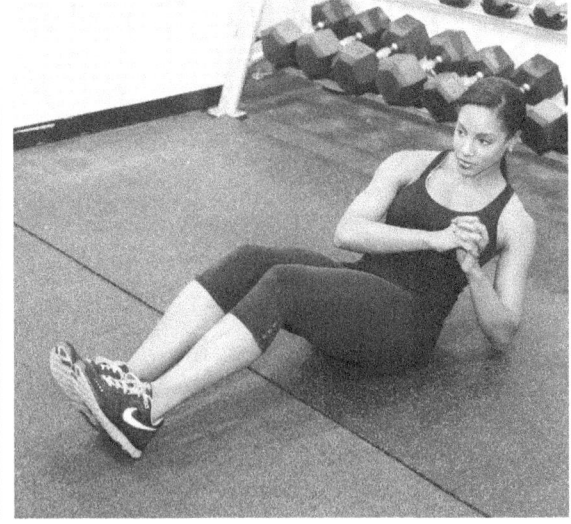

RUSSIAN TWIST

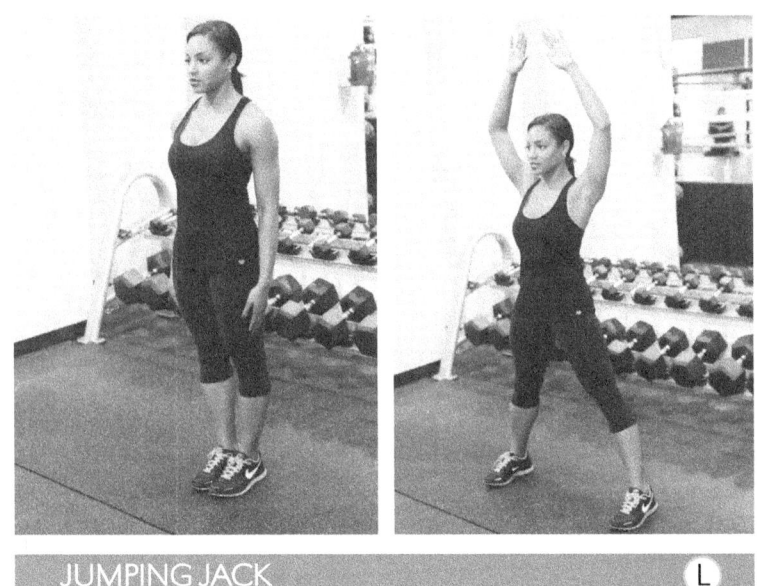

JUMPING JACK

WORKOUT JOURNAL LIGHT DAYS

WEEK 1

WEEK 2

WEEK 3

WEEK 4

WEEKS 1 THROUGH 4 ONLY

MODERATE DAY: 25 MINUTE WORKOUT

5 x 15 x 5 ROUTINE

(5 Exercises x 15 Repetitions x 5 Sets)

Sumo Squat

Dip

Reverse Lunge (Step Backward - 15 each leg)

Plank with Knees to Chest (Hold plank and alternate knees to chest)

Squat Jump

***Perform the five exercises in the set with the given amount of repetitions.
Rest one minute then repeat until the five sets are completed.***

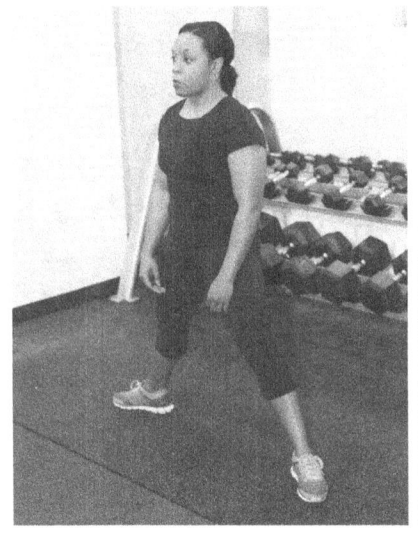
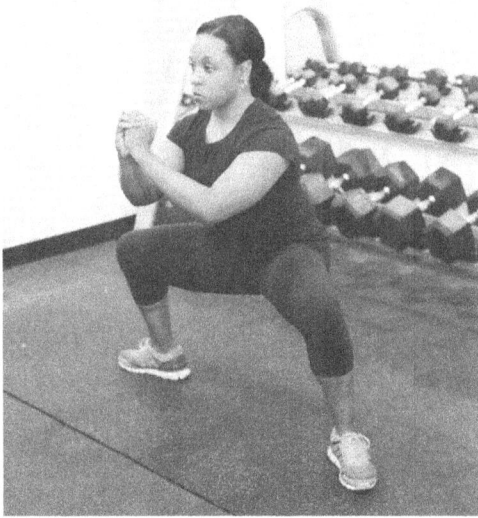

SUMO SQUAT

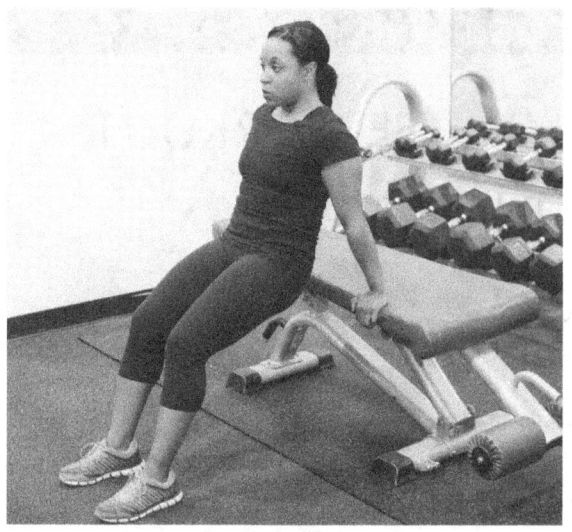
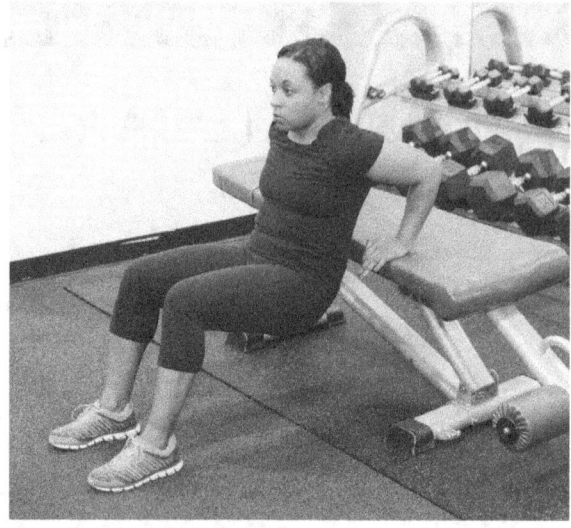

DIP

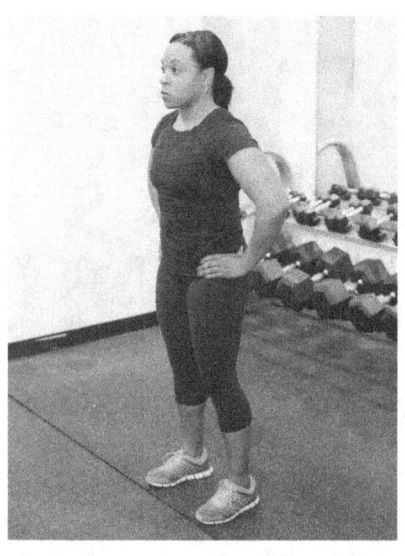
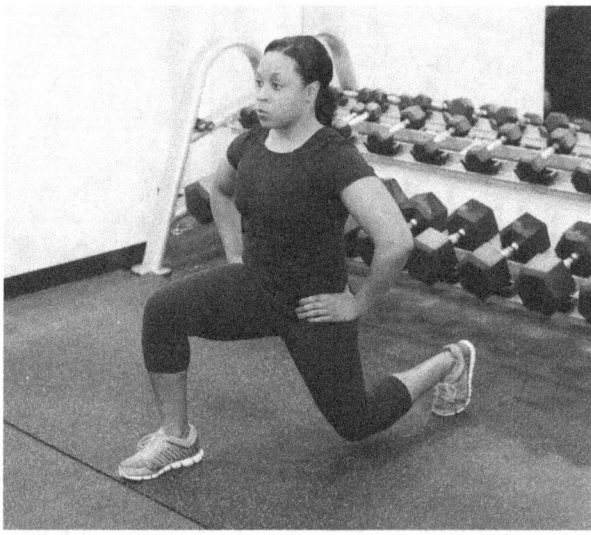

REVERSE LUNGE

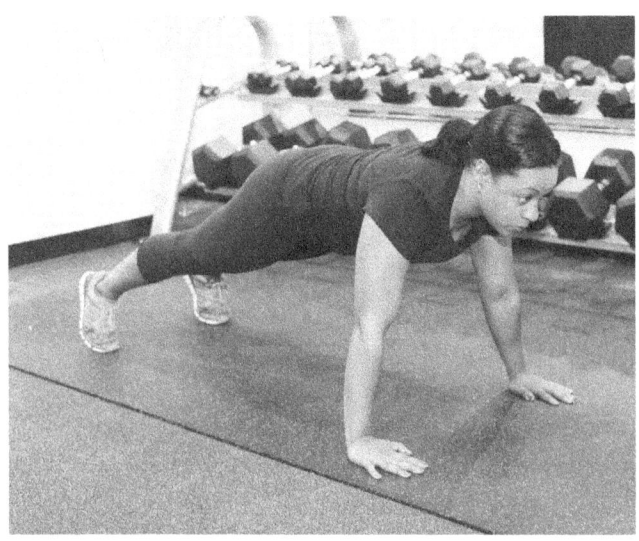
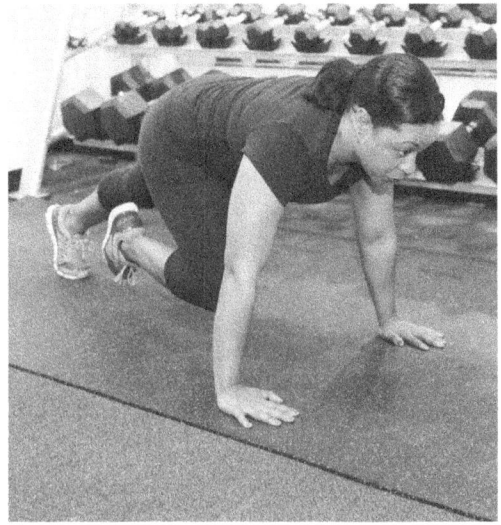

PLANK WITH KNEES TO CHEST

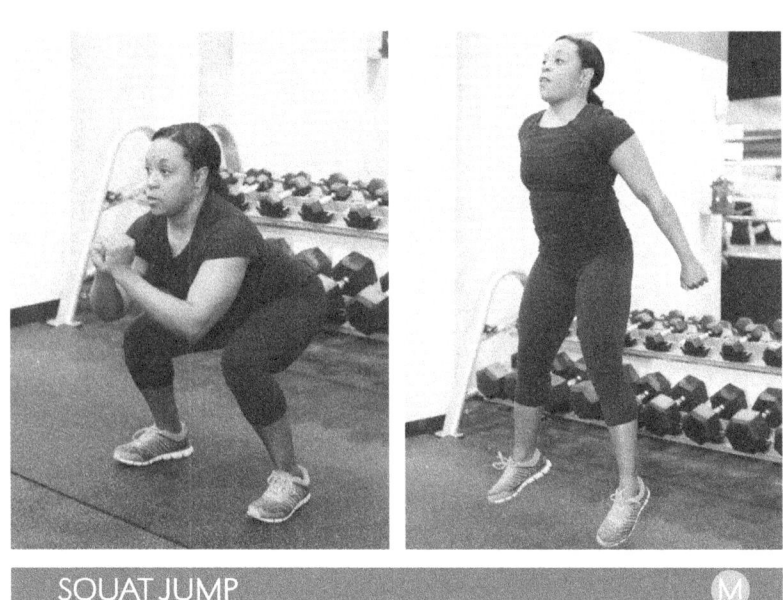

SQUAT JUMP

WORKOUT JOURNAL MODERATE DAYS

WEEK 1

WEEK 2

WEEK 3

WEEK 4

WEEKS 1 THROUGH 4 ONLY

HARD DAY: 30 MINUTE WORKOUT

5 x 20 x 5 ROUTINE
(5 Exercises x 20 Repetitions x 5 Sets)
Squat
Push-Up
Forward Lunge (Step forward - 20 each leg))
Sit Up
Burpee

***Perform the five exercises in the set with the given amount of repetitions.
Rest one to two minutes then repeat until the five sets are completed.***

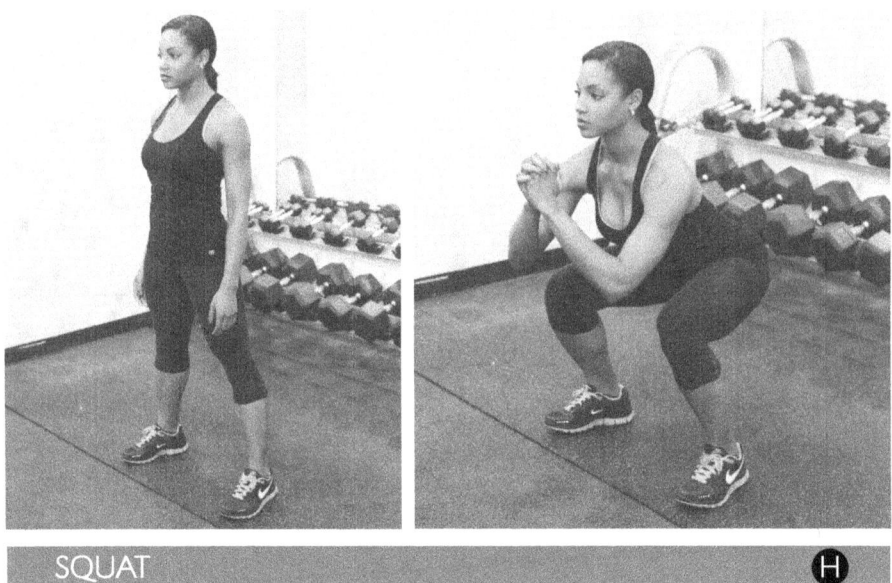

SQUAT

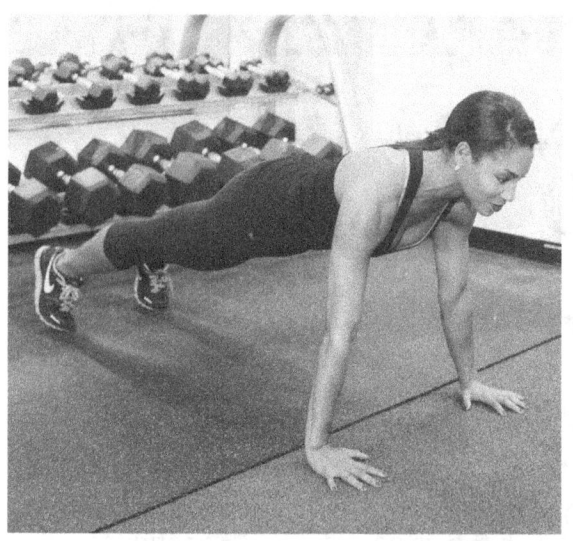
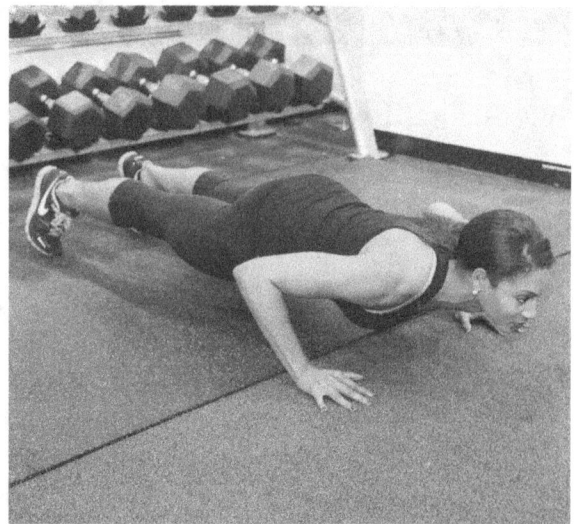

PUSH-UP

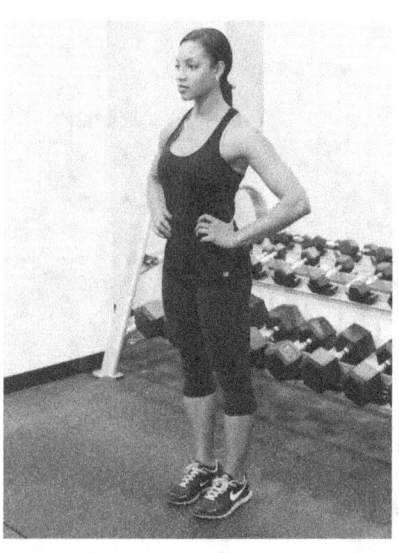
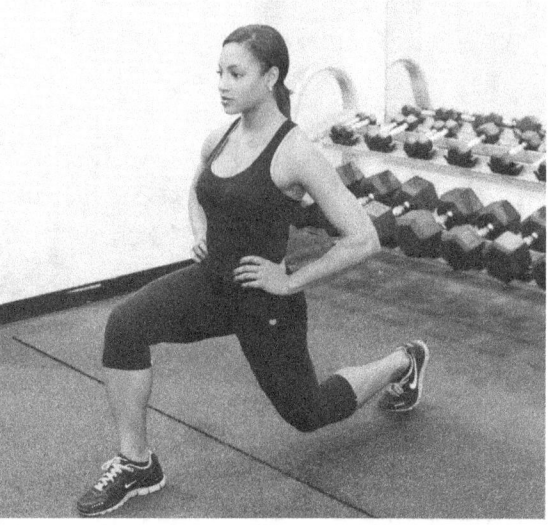

FORWARD LUNGE

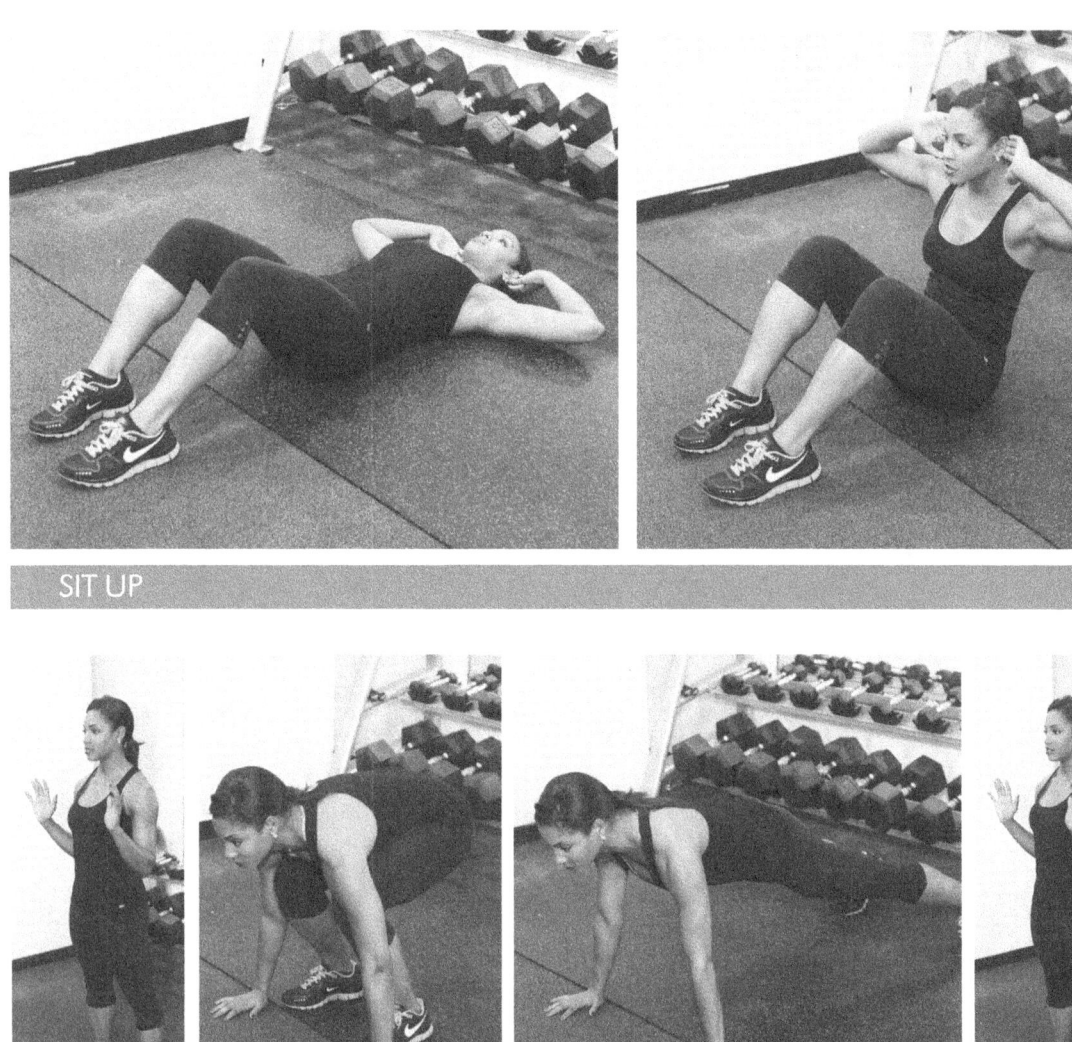

SIT UP

BURPEE

WORKOUT JOURNAL HARD DAYS

WEEK 1

WEEK 2

WEEK 3

WEEK 4

YOU'VE COMPLETED 4 WEEKS:

Current Weight _____ Date _____

- What Goals have I reached in the past 4 weeks?

_____

_____

_____

- What is my reward for reaching these goals?

_____

_____

_____

- Have I done my best to uphold my contract?

_____

_____

_____

- What challenges did I face in the last 4 weeks and what did I do to overcome them?

_____

_____

_____

- What are potential personal and fitness challenges that I may face in the next 4 weeks?

- What are things I can do to prepare to make the next 4 weeks of training better?

WEEK 5 CHALLENGE:
5 DAY PLANK CHALLENGE
(End of Week 4- Perform 5 consecutive days in addition to
scheduled workouts in Week 5)

DAY 1	DAY 2	DAY 3	DAY 4	DAY 5
Plank = 30 Sec	Plank = 45 Sec	Plank = 1 Min	Plank = 1:15 Min	Plank = 1:30 Min

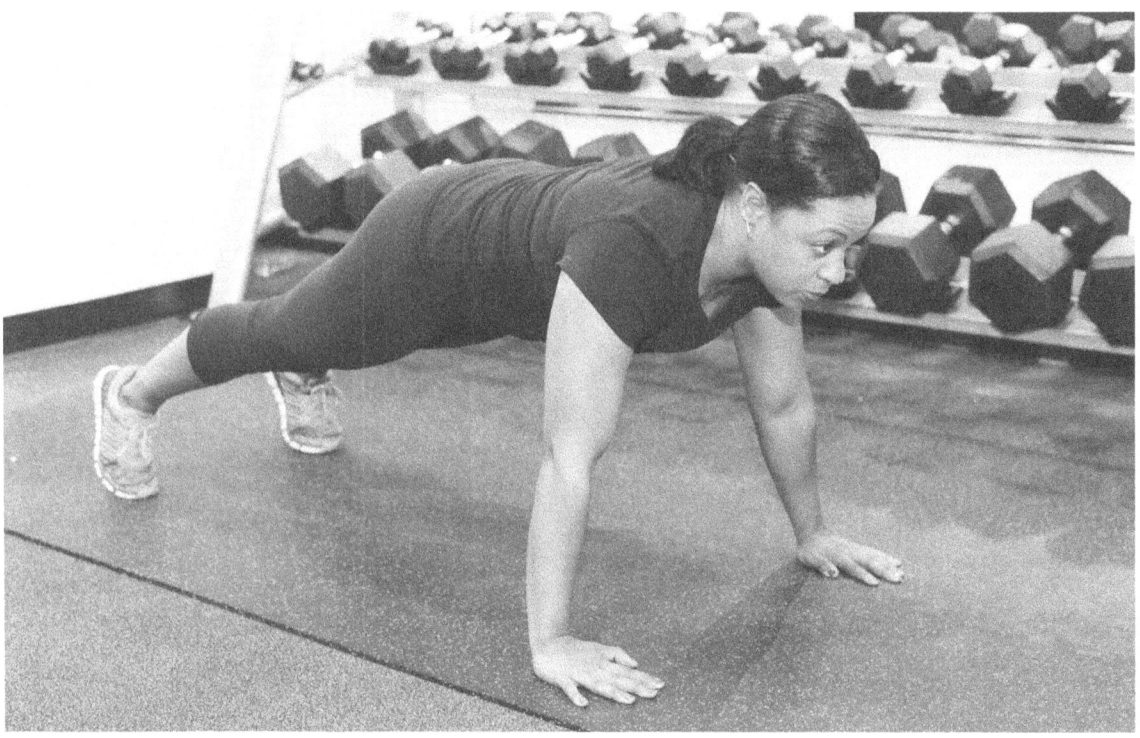

PLANK

WEEKS 5 THROUGH 8 ONLY

LIGHT DAY: 20 MINUTE WORKOUT

5 x 10 x 5 ROUTINE
(5 Exercises x 10 Repetitions x 5 Sets)
Hip Abduction with band (10 each leg)
Push-Up
Bicycle Crunch (10 each leg)
Overhead Tricep Extension (w/ band or dumbbells)
Speed Skater (10 each leg)
***Perform the five exercises in the set with the given amount of repetitions.
Rest thirty seconds to one minute then repeat until the five sets are completed.***

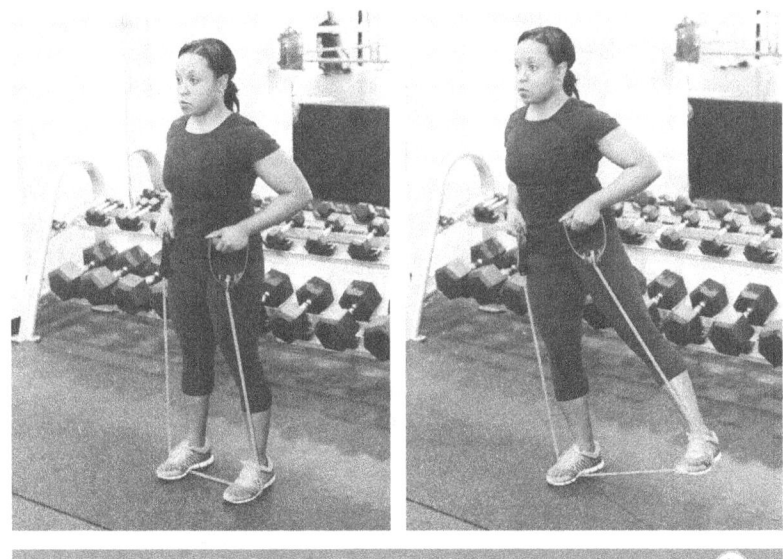

HIP ABDUCTION WITH BAND ⓛ

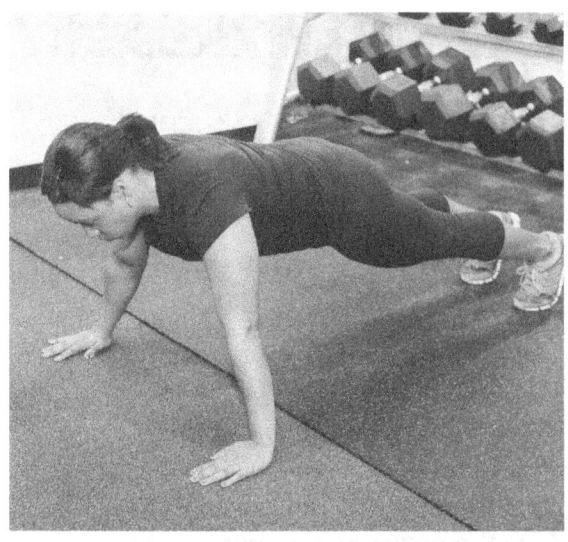 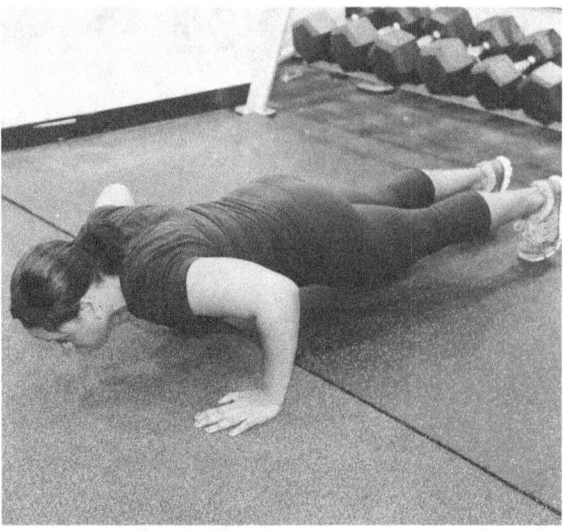

PUSH-UP (L)

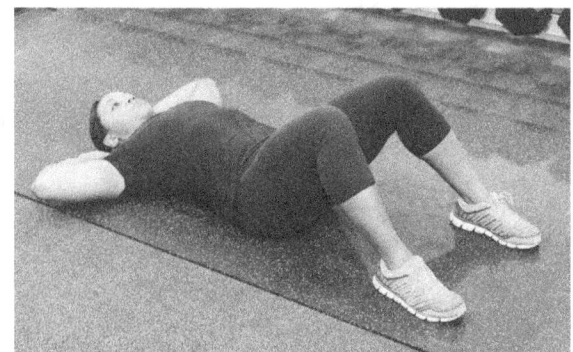 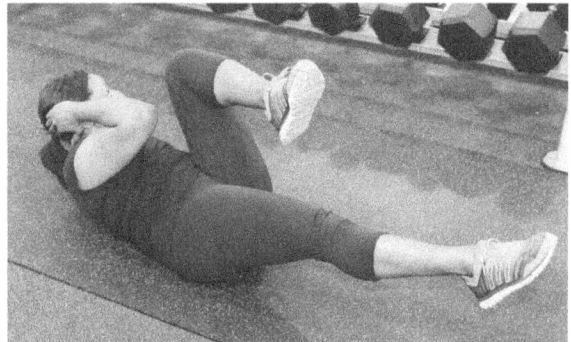

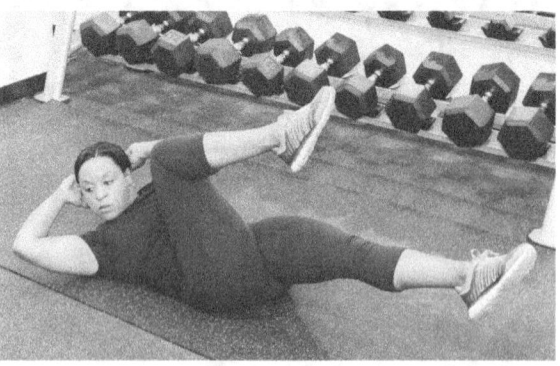

BICYCLE CRUNCH (L)

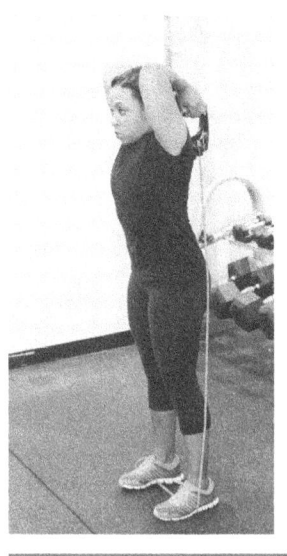 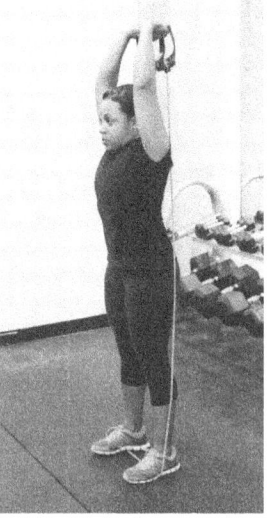 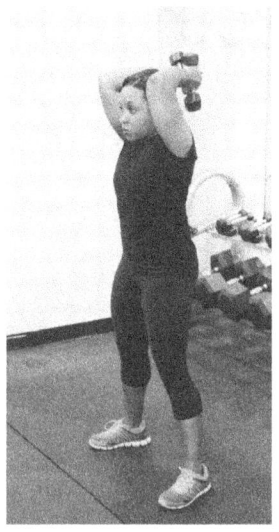 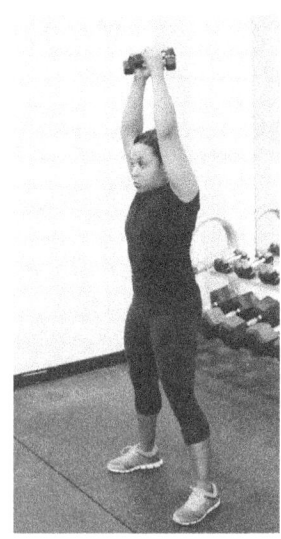

OVERHEAD TRICEP EXTENSION (W/ BAND OR DUMBBELLS)   L

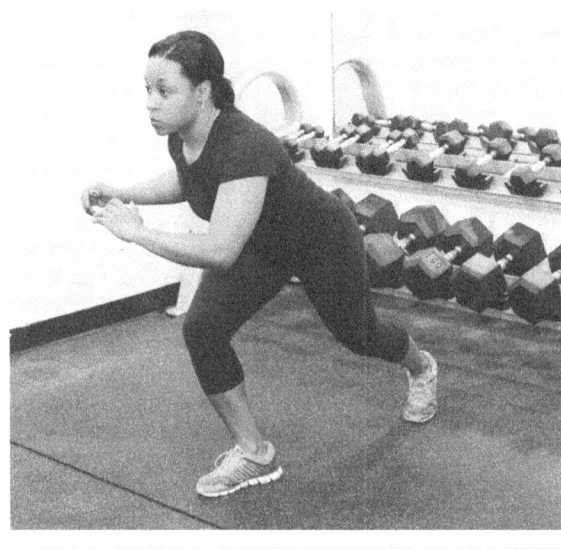 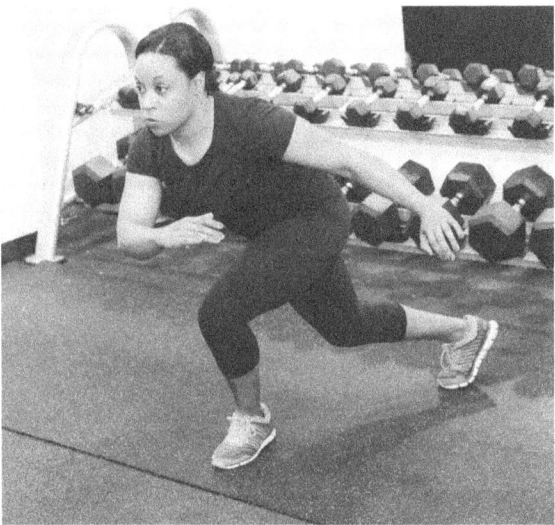

SPEED SKATER   L

WORKOUT JOURNAL LIGHT DAYS

WEEK 5

WEEK 6

WEEK 7

WEEK 8

WEEKS 5 THROUGH 8 ONLY

MODERATE DAY: 25 MINUTE WORKOUT

5 x 15 x 5 ROUTINE
(5 Exercises x 15 Repetitions x 5 Sets)
Squat
Double Arm Row (w/band or dumbbells)
Suitcase Crunch
Side Lunge (15 each leg)
Quick Mountain Climber (15 each leg)
(Hold plank and move knees to chest in a running motion)
***Perform the five exercises in the set with the given amount of repetitions.
Rest one minute then repeat until the five sets are completed.***

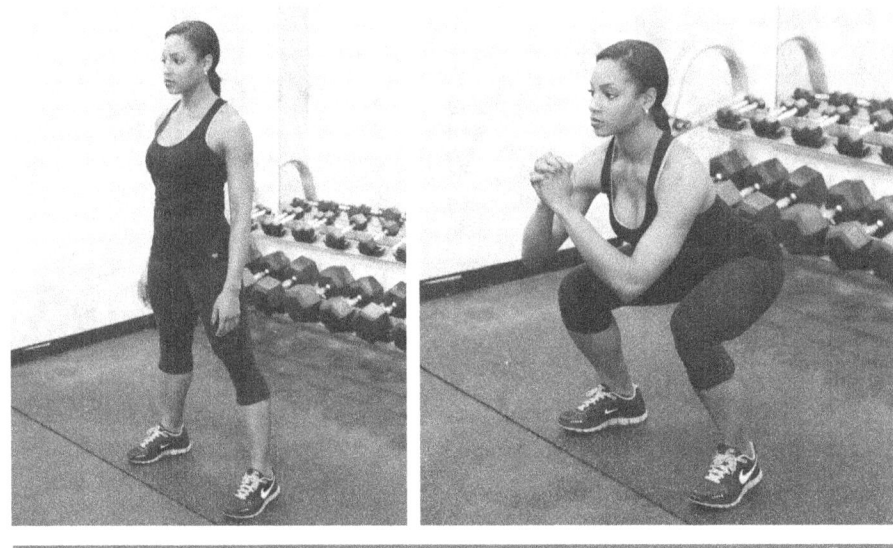

SQUAT

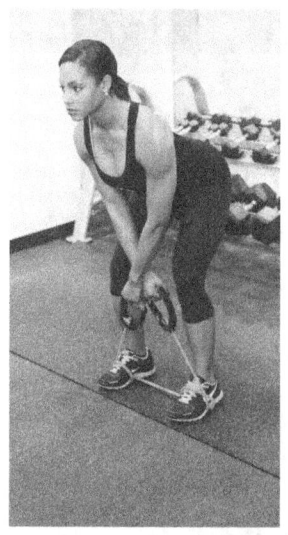 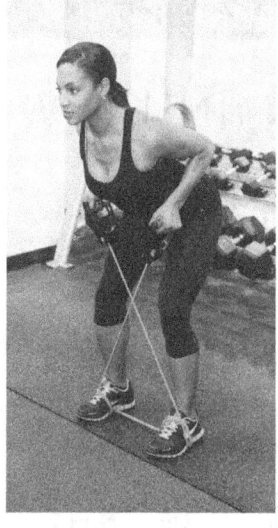 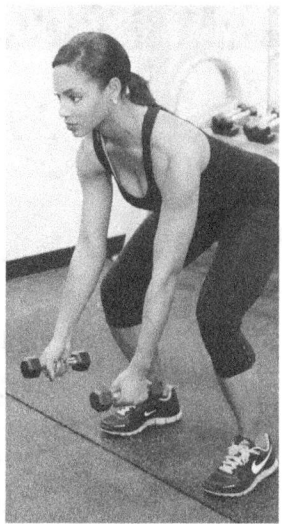 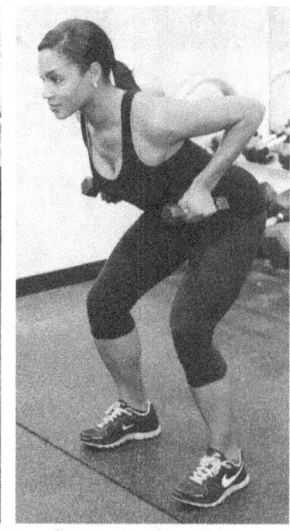

DOUBLE ARM ROW (W/BAND OR DUMBBELLS)

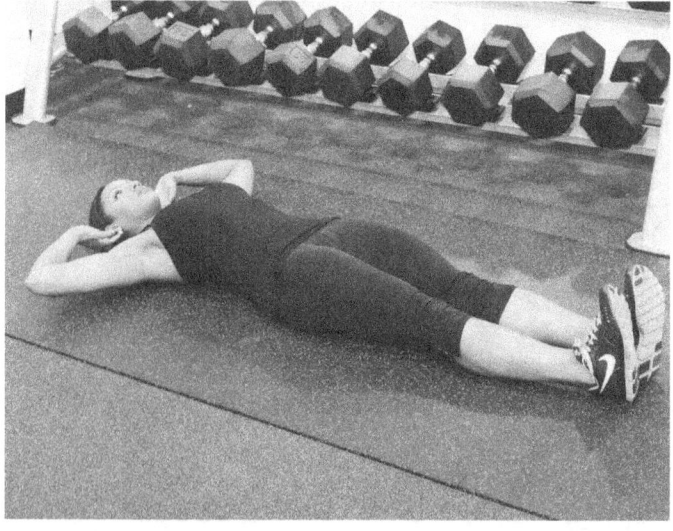 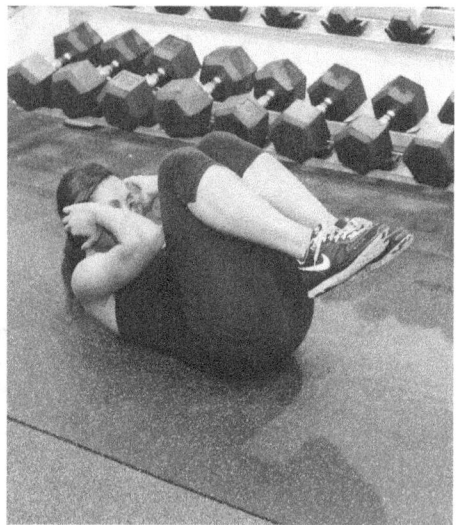

SUITCASE CRUNCH

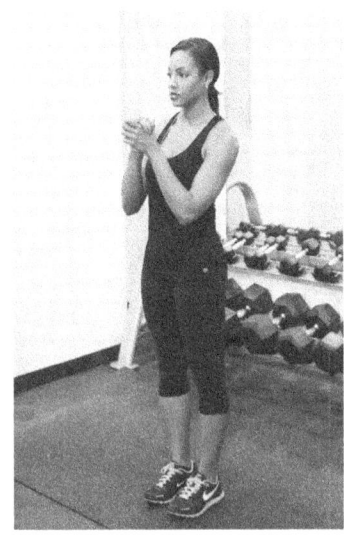
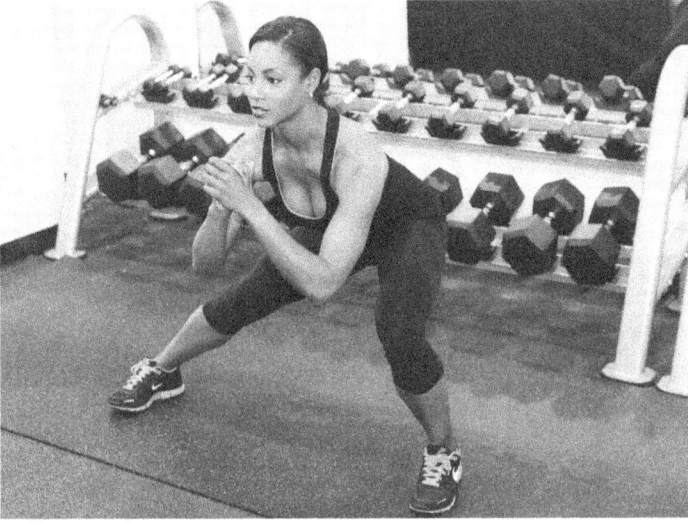

SIDE LUNGE

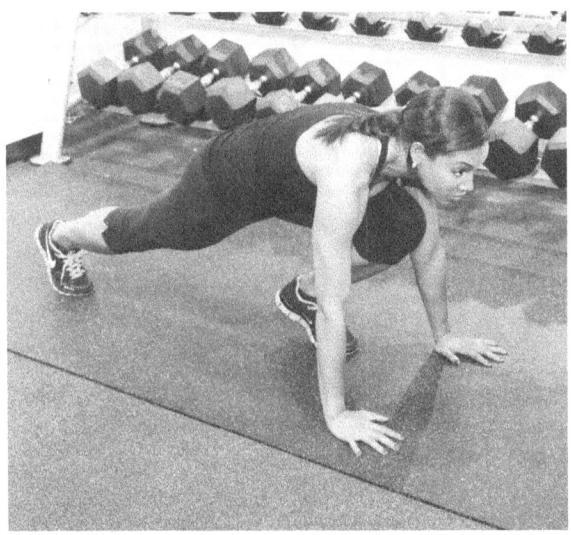
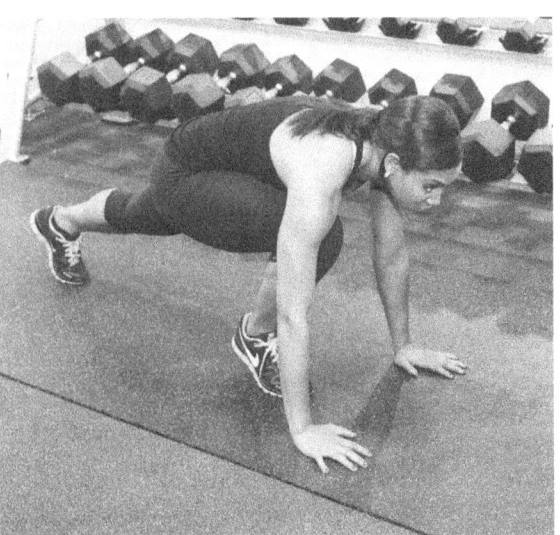

QUICK MOUNTAIN CLIMBER

WORKOUT JOURNAL MODERATE DAYS

WEEK 5

WEEK 6

WEEK 7

WEEK 8

WEEKS 5 THROUGH 8 ONLY

HARD DAY: 30 MINUTE WORKOUT

5 x 20 x 5 ROUTINE
(5 Exercises x 20 Repetitions x 5 Sets)
Forward Lunge (Step forward - 20 each leg)
Shoulder Press (w/ band or dumbbells)
Leg Drop-Lift
Bicep Curl (w/ band or dumbbells)
Burpee with Push-Up
***Perform the five exercises in the set with the given amount of repetitions.
Rest one to two minutes then repeat until the five sets are completed.***

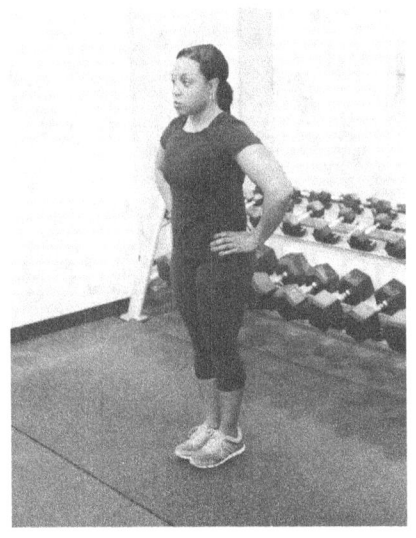 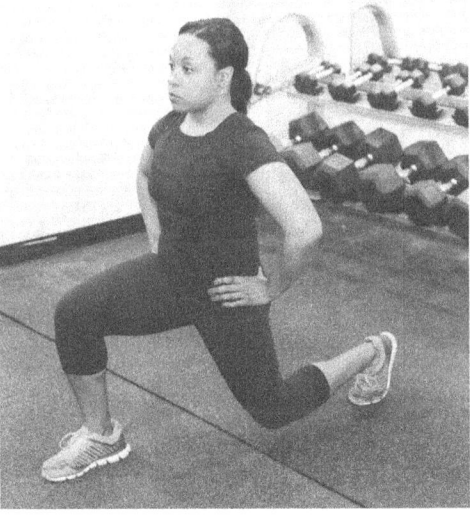

FORWARD LUNGE

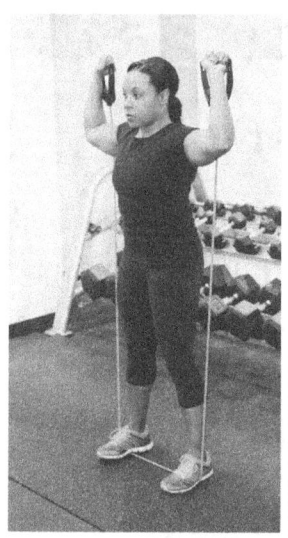 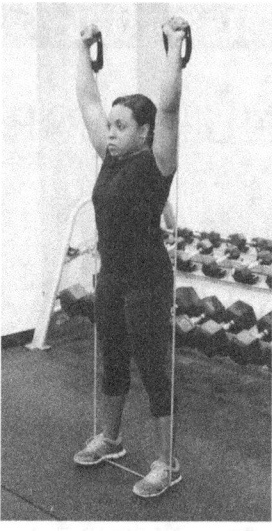 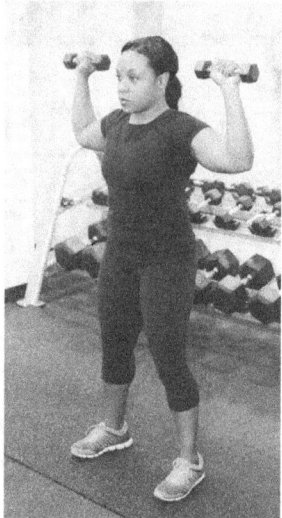 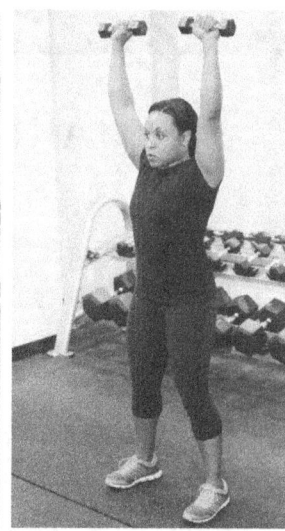

SHOULDER PRESS (W/ BAND OR DUMBBELLS)

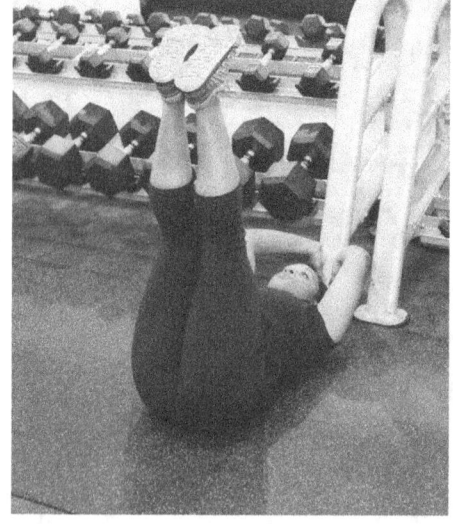 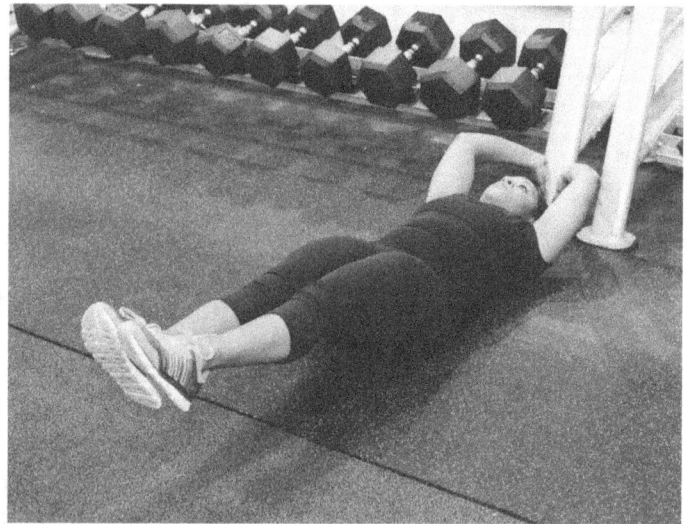

LEG DROP-LIFT

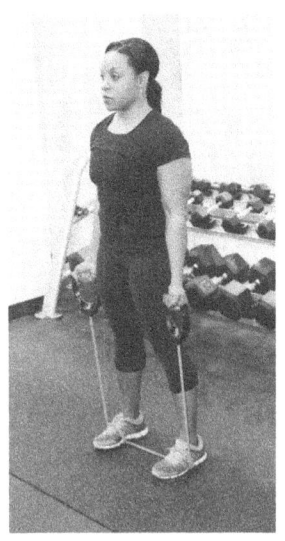 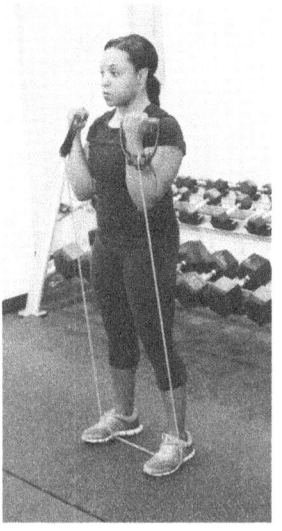 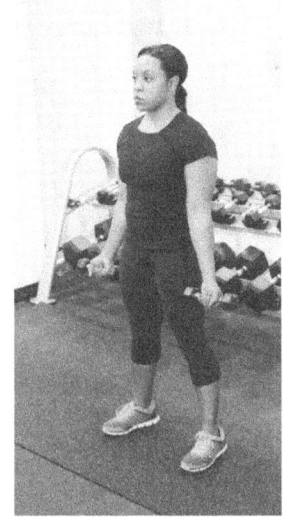 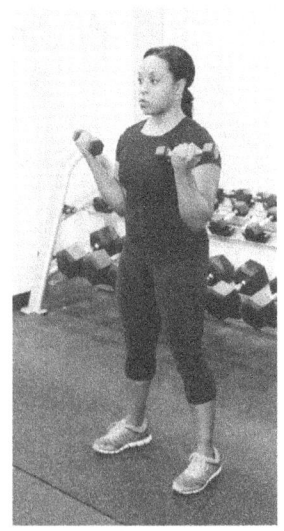

BICEP CURL (W/ BAND OR DUMBBELLS)

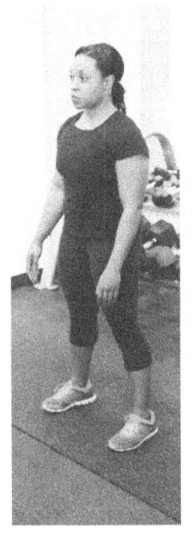 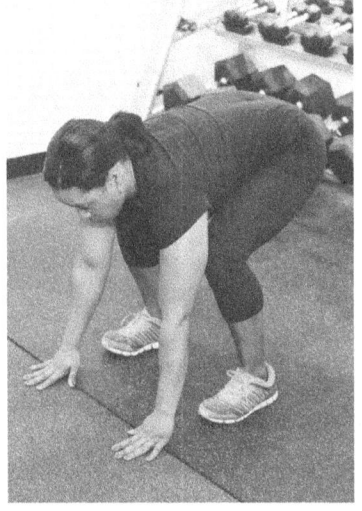 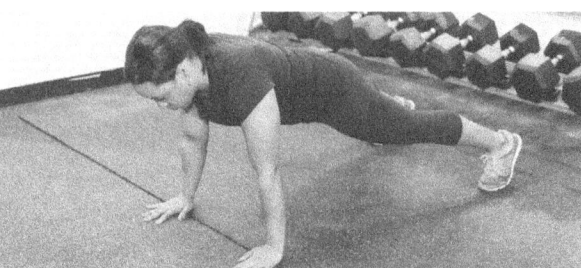

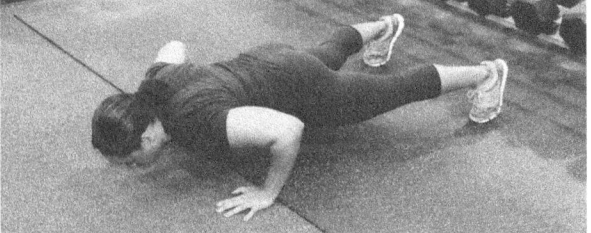

BURPEE WITH PUSH-UP

WORKOUT JOURNAL HARD DAYS

WEEK 5

WEEK 6

WEEK 7

WEEK 8

YOU'VE COMPLETED 8 WEEKS

Current Weight _____ Date _____

- What Goals have I reached in the past 8 weeks?

_____

_____

_____

_____

- What is my reward for reaching these goals?

_____

_____

_____

_____

- Have I done my best to uphold my contract?

_____

_____

_____

_____

- What challenges did I face in the last 8 weeks and what did I do to overcome them?

_____

_____

_____

_____

• What are potential personal and fitness challenges that I may face in the next 4 weeks?

_____

_____

_____

_____

• What are things I can do to prepare to make the last 4 weeks of training better?

_____

_____

_____

_____

WEEK 9 CHALLENGE:
5 DAY SQUAT CHALLENGE
(End of Week 8 and Perform 5 consecutive days in addition to
scheduled workouts in Week 9)

DAY 1	DAY 2	DAY 3	DAY 4	DAY 5
20 Squats	40 Squats	60 Squats	80 Squats	100 Squats

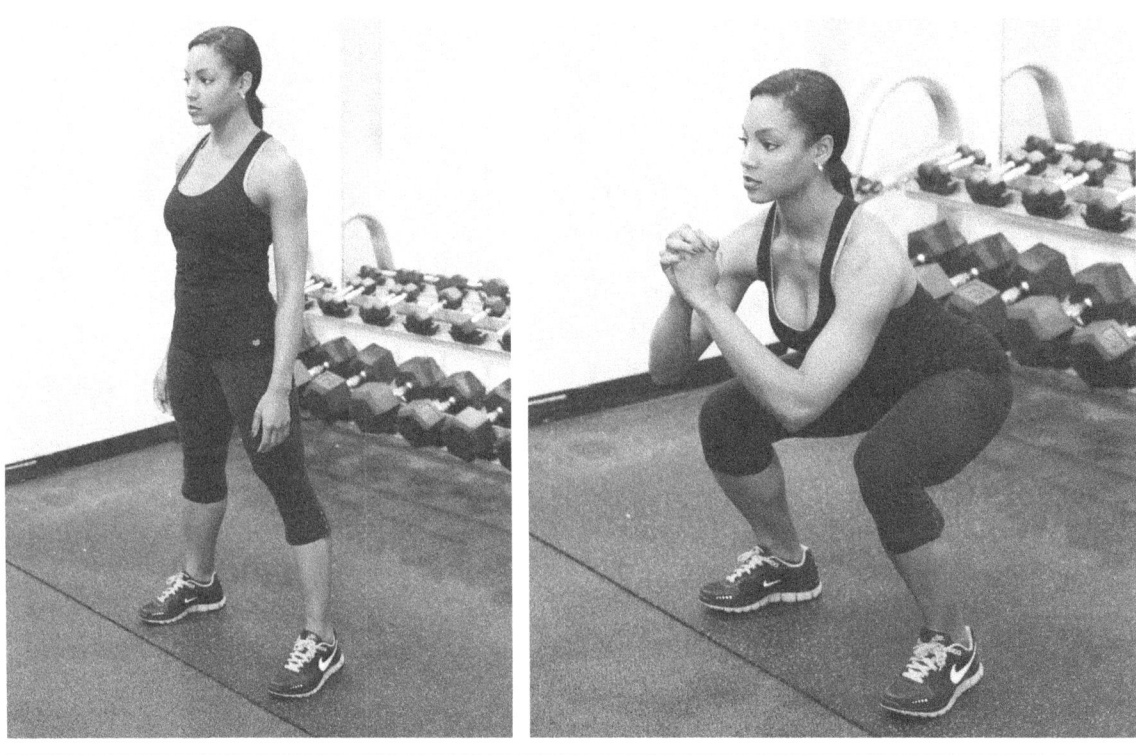

SQUAT

LIGHT DAY: 20 MINUTE WORKOUT

5 x 10 x 5 ROUTINE

(5 Exercises x 10 Repetitions x 5 Sets)
Sumo Squat (w/ band or dumbbells)
Chest Press (w/band or dumbbells)
Bridge
Palms Down Bicep Curl (w/ band or dumbbells)
Plank Jack (Hold plank and move legs in jumping jack motion)
***Perform the five exercises in the set with the given amount of repetitions.
Rest thirty seconds to one minute then repeat until the five sets are completed.***

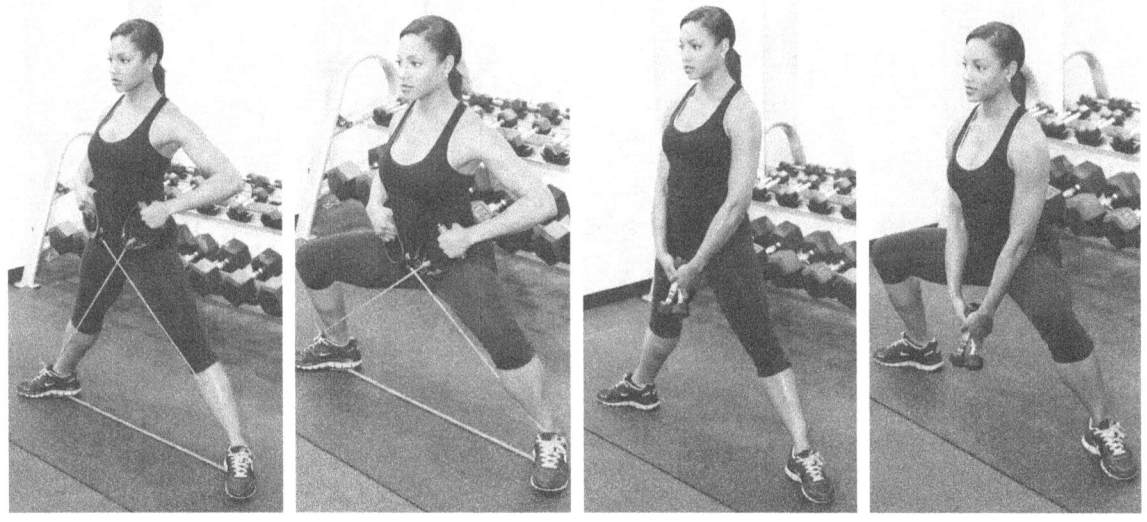

SUMO SQUAT (W/ BAND OR DUMBBELLS)   L

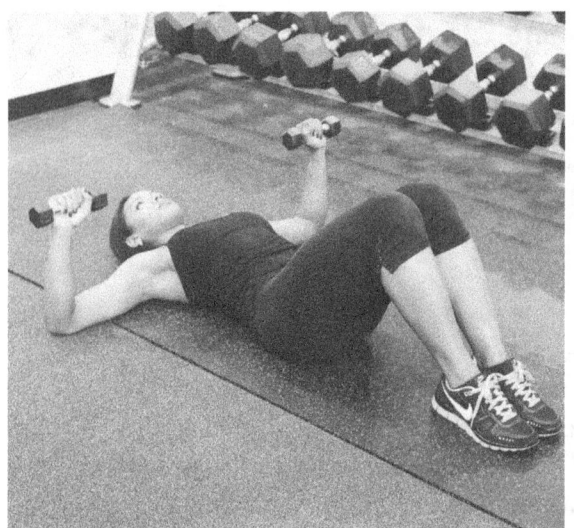 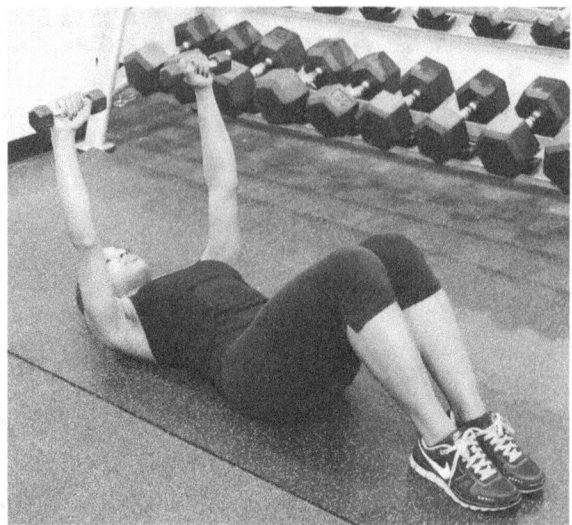

CHEST PRESS WITH DUMBBELLS (L)

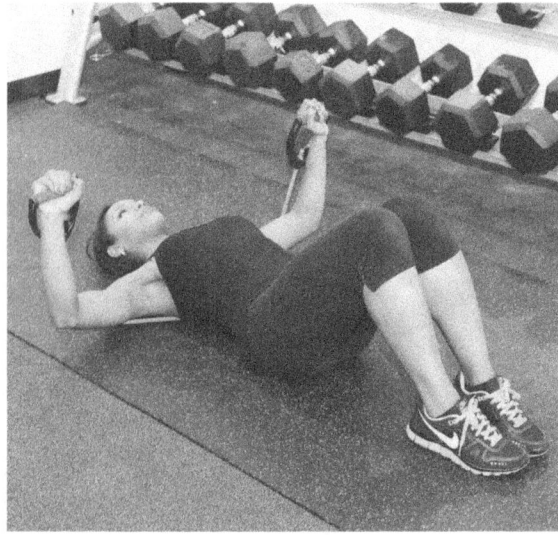 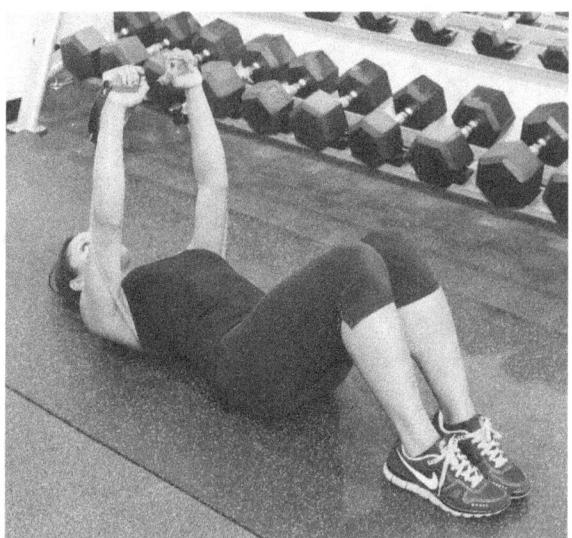

CHEST PRESS WITH BAND OPTION (L)

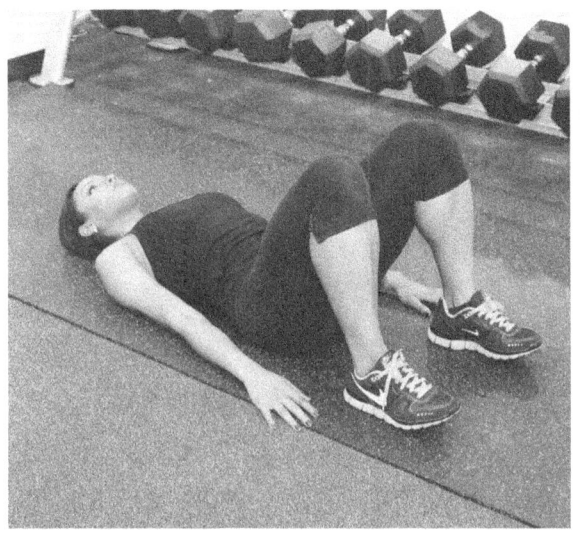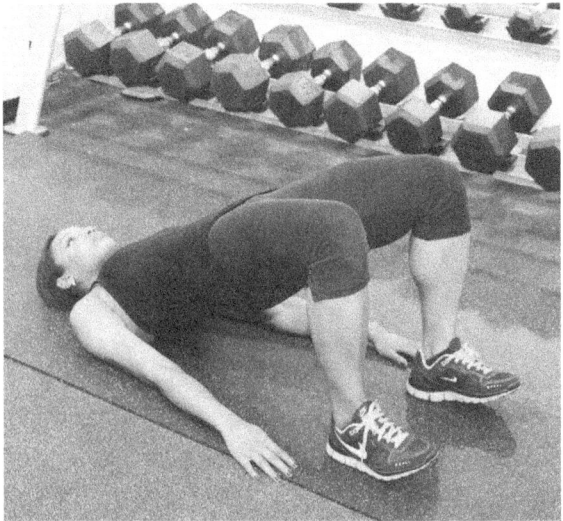

BRIDGE

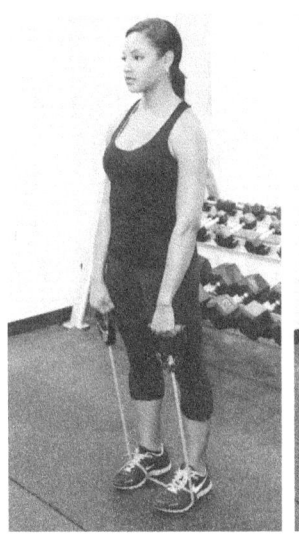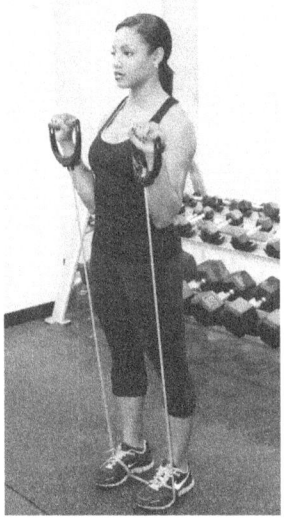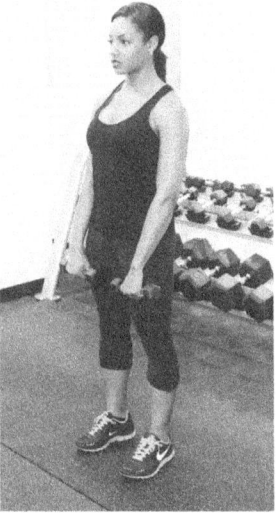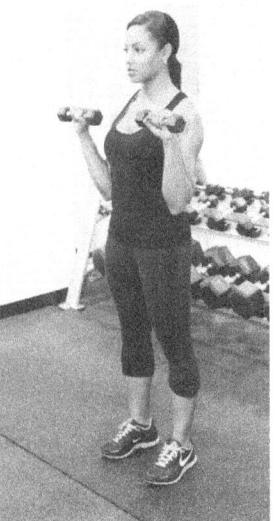

PALMS DOWN BICEP CURLS (W/ BAND OR DUMBBELLS)

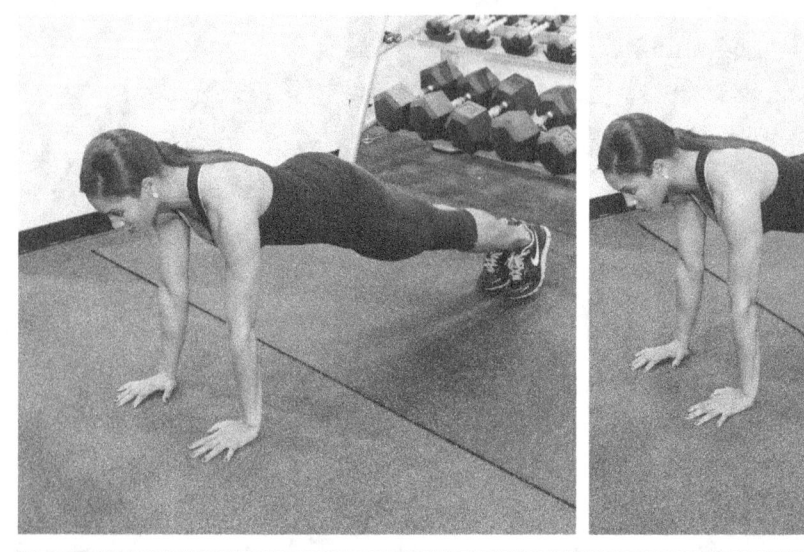

PLANK JACK

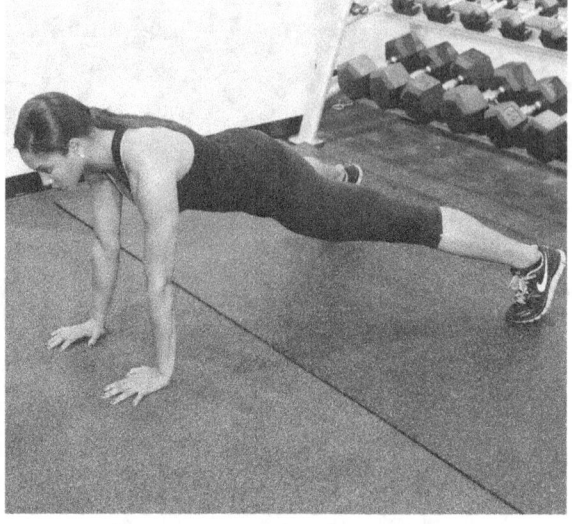

L

WORKOUT JOURNAL LIGHT DAYS

WEEK 9

WEEK 10

WEEK 11

WEEK 12

WEEKS 9 THROUGH 12 ONLY

MODERATE DAY: 25 MINUTE WORKOUT

5 x 15 x 5 ROUTINE

(5 Exercises x 15 Repetitions x 5 Sets = 75 Total Reps per Exercise)
Diagonal Forward Lunge (Step forward diagonally - 15 each leg)
Frontal Raise (w/band or dumbbells)
Dip
Woodchopper
Pike Jump (Hold plank and jump legs in and back out into plank)
***Perform the five exercises in the set with the given amount of repetitions.
Rest one minute then repeat until the five sets are completed.***

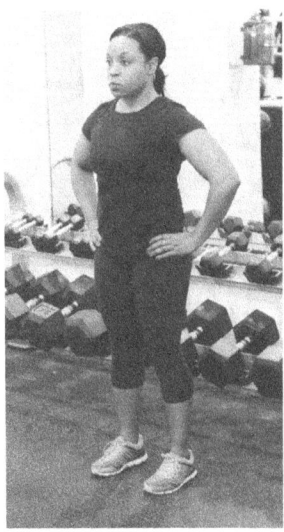 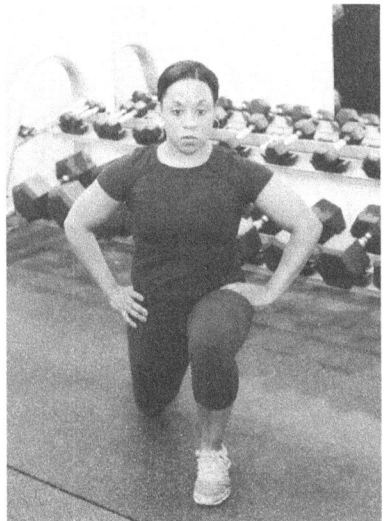 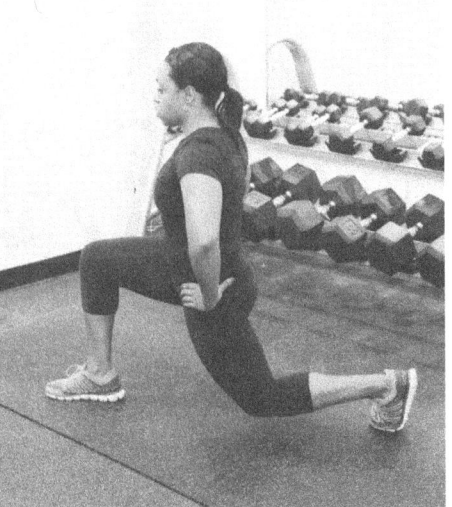

DIAGONAL FORWARD LUNGE

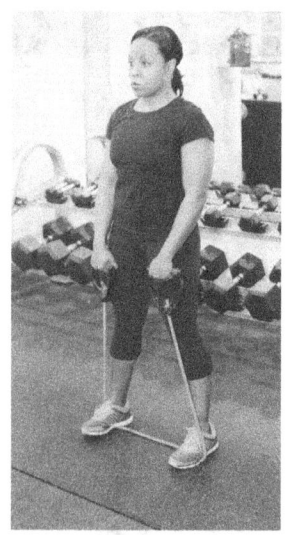 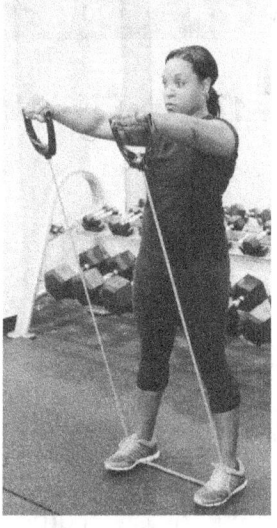 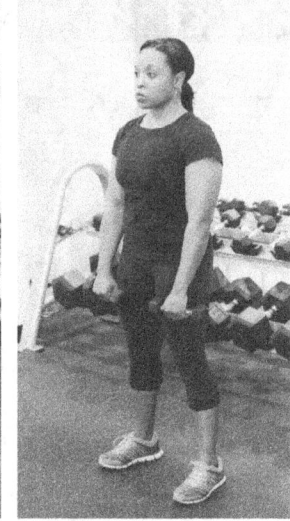 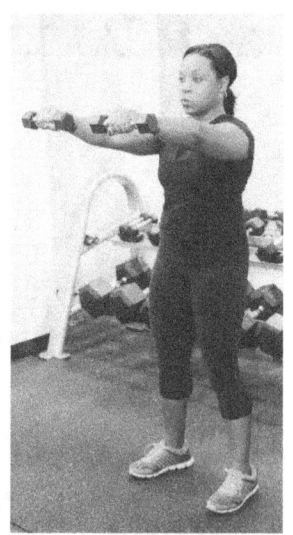

FRONTAL RAISE (W/BAND OR DUMBBELLS)

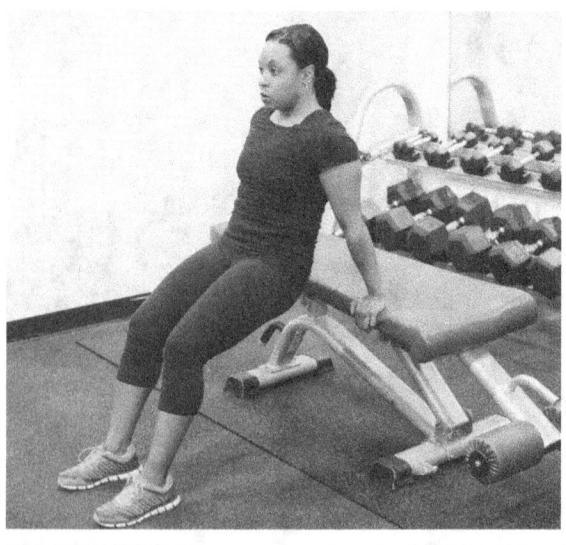 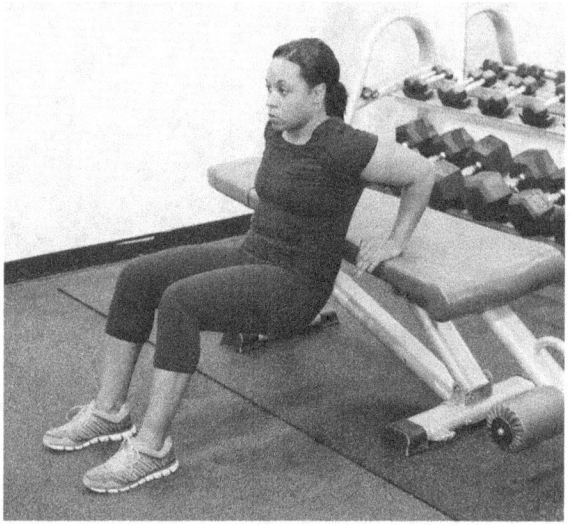

DIP

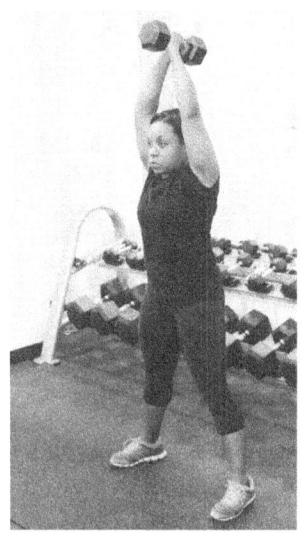
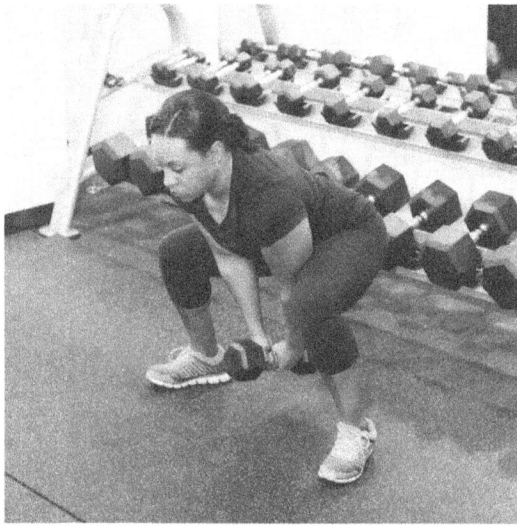
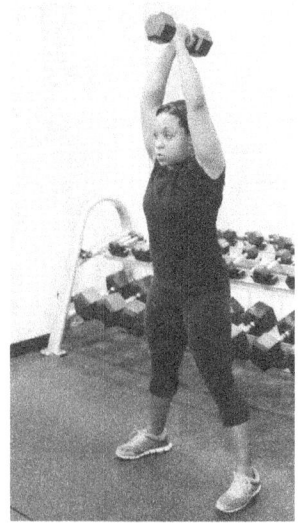

WOODCHOPPER

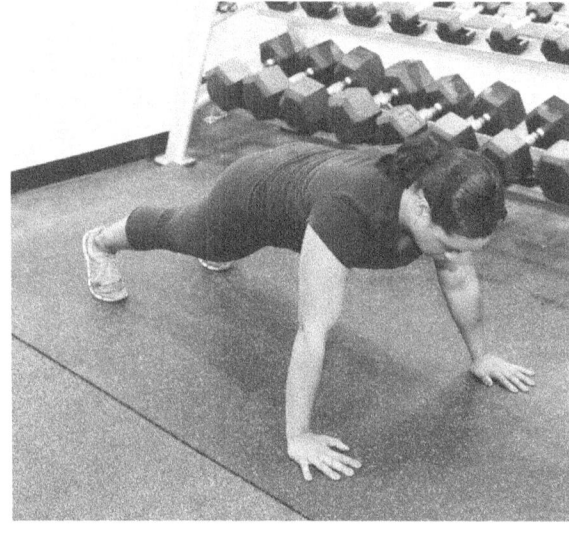
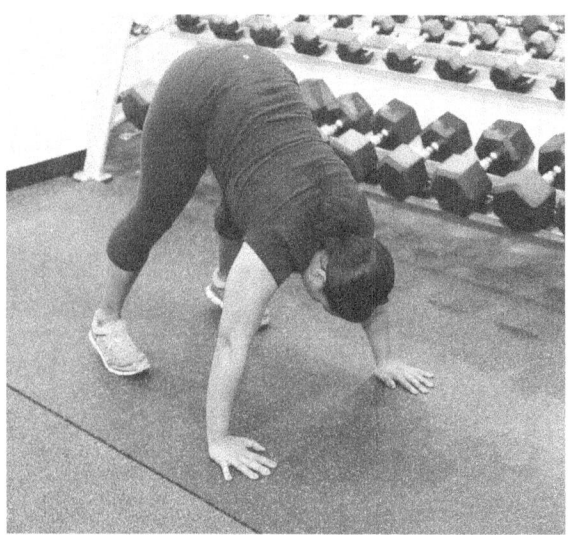

PIKE JUMP

WORKOUT JOURNAL MODERATE DAYS

WEEK 9

WEEK 10

WEEK 11

WEEK 12

WEEKS 9 THROUGH 12 ONLY

HARD DAY: 30 MINUTE WORKOUT

5 x 20 x 5 ROUTINE

(5 Exercises x 20 Repetitions x 5 Sets)

Split Squat (Start in split stance and lower and lift your body - 20 each leg)
Arnold Press (w/ band or dumbbells)
Reverse Fly (w/band or dumbbells)
Plank w/ Opposite Knee to Opposite Elbow (20 each leg)
Side to Side Squat Jump (Squat Jump left then Squat Jump right)
***Perform the five exercises in the set with the given amount of repetitions.
Rest one to two minutes then repeat until the five sets are completed.***

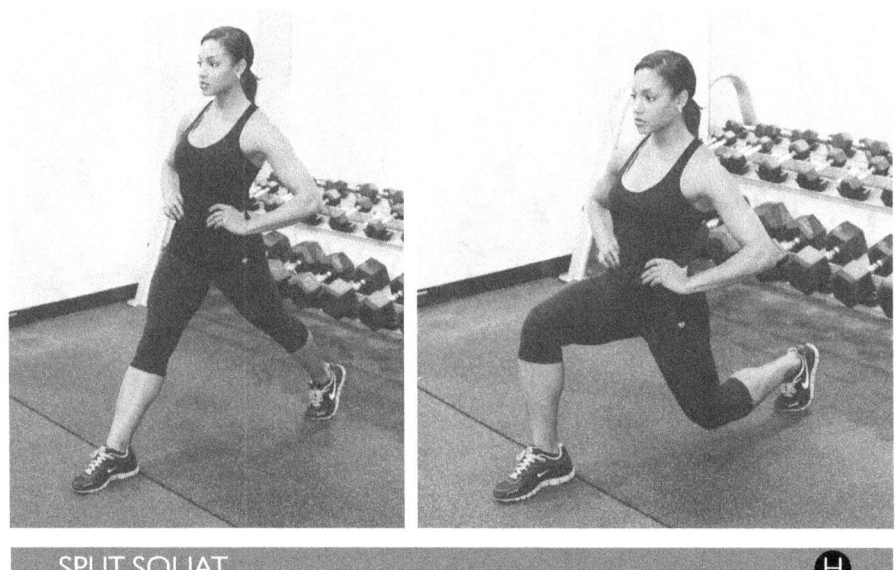

SPLIT SQUAT

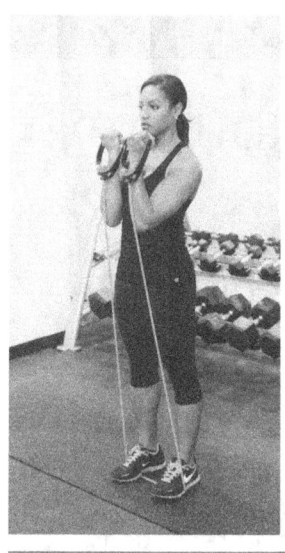 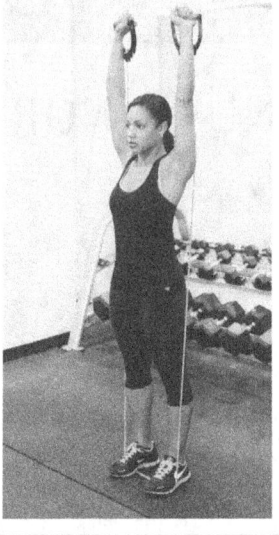 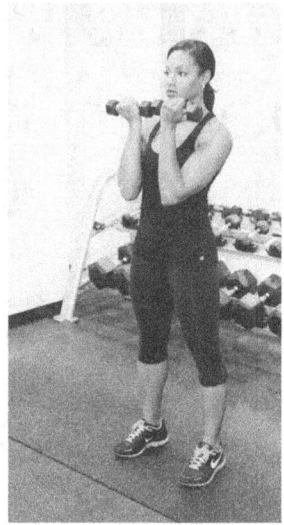 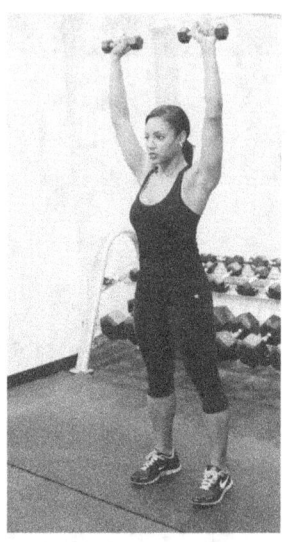

ARNOLD PRESS (W/ BAND OR DUMBBELLS)

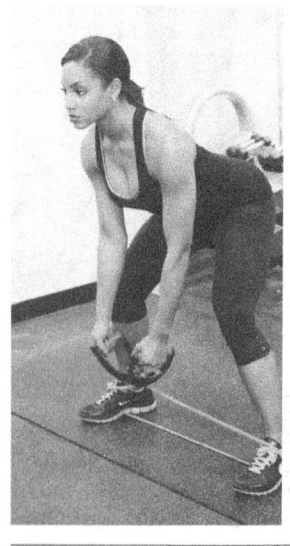 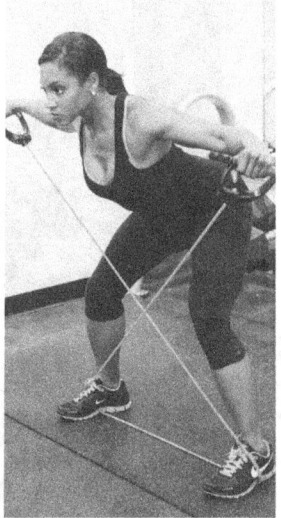 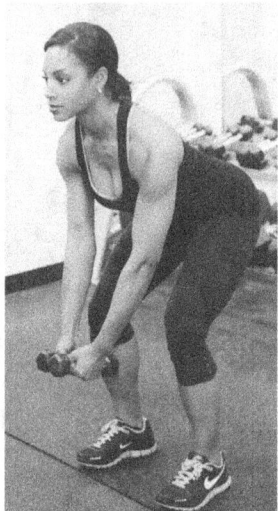 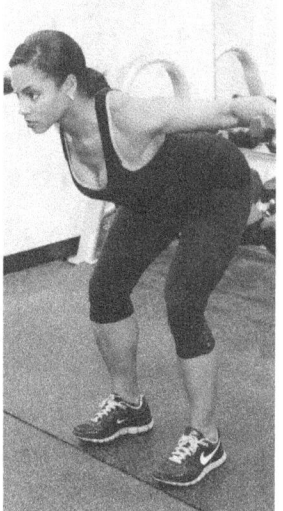

REVERSE FLY (W/BAND OR DUMBBELLS)

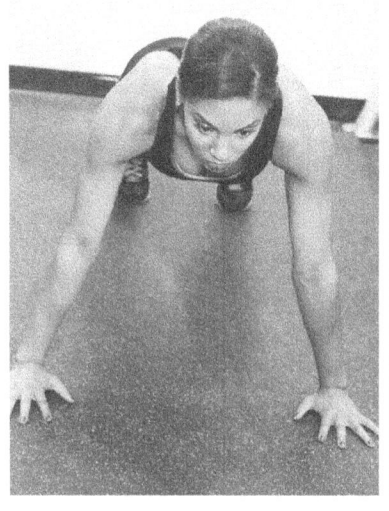 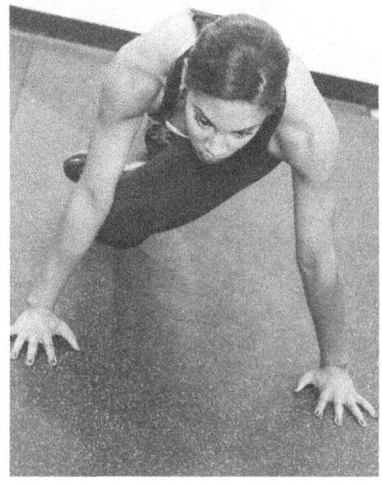 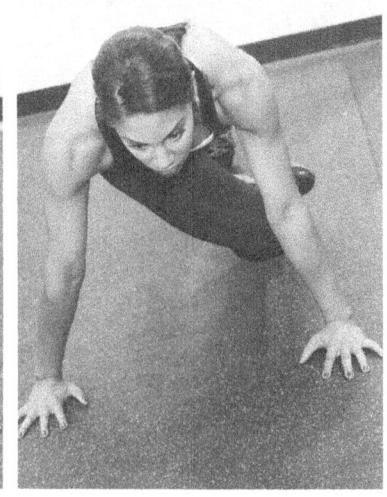

PLANK W/ OPPOSITE KNEE TO OPPOSITE ELBOW

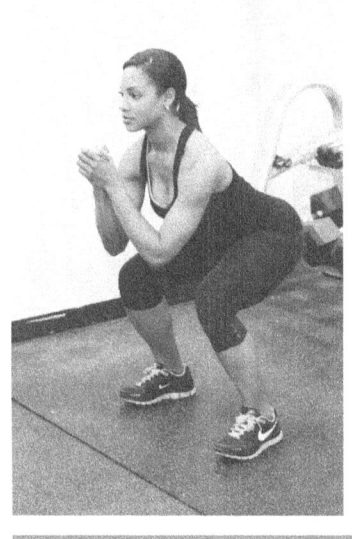 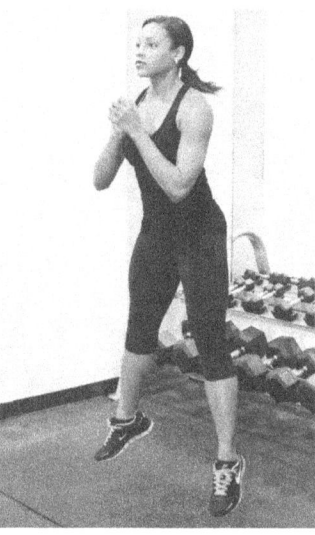 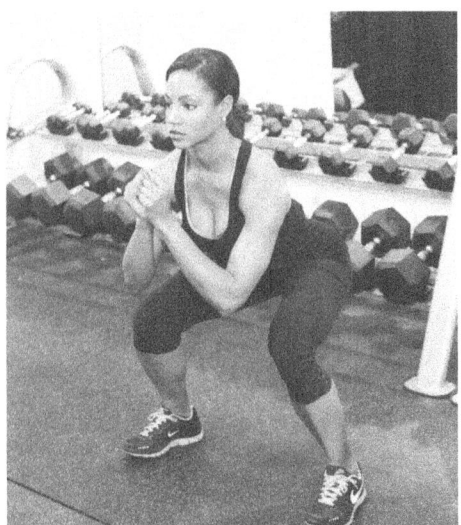

SIDE TO SIDE SQUAT JUMP

WORKOUT JOURNAL HARD DAYS

WEEK 9 _____

_____

_____

_____

WEEK 10 _____

_____

_____

_____

WEEK 11 _____

_____

_____

_____

WEEK 12 _____

_____

_____

_____

WEEK 12 CHALLENGE:
5 DAY BURPEE CHALLENGE
(Perform 5 consecutive days)

DAY 1	DAY 2	DAY 3	DAY 4	DAY 5
10 Burpees	15 Burpees	20 Burpees	25 Burpees	30 Burpees

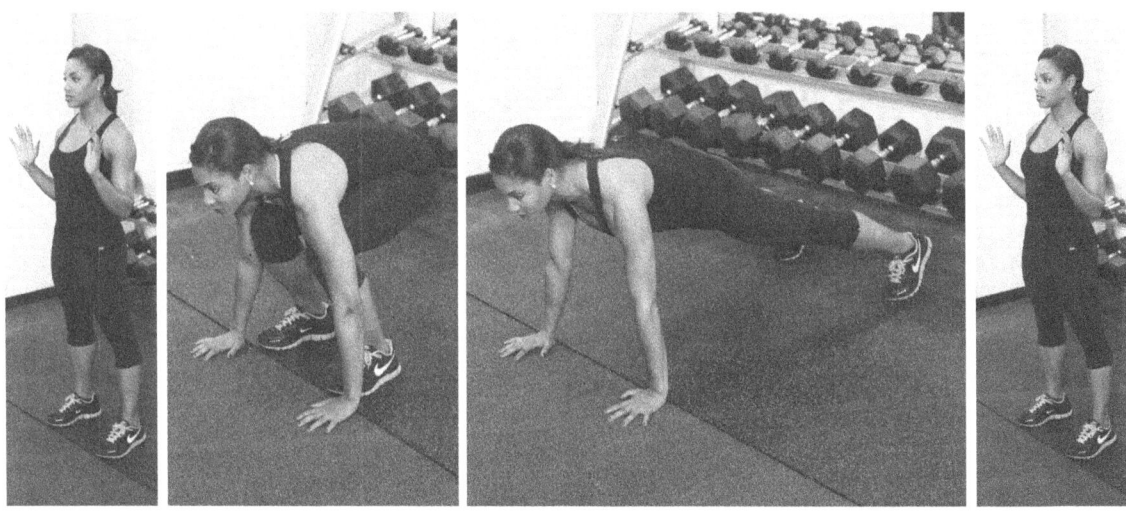

BURPEE

YOU'VE COMPLETED 12 WEEKS!

Ending Weight _____   Date _____

- What Short-Term Goals have I achieved over the last 12 weeks?

  _____

  _____

  _____

- What Intermediate Goals have I achieved over the last 12 weeks?

  _____

  _____

  _____

- What do I still need to do to fulfill my Long-Term Goals?

  _____

  _____

  _____

- Do my Ultimate Goals still feel realistic and attainable?

  _____

  _____

  _____

- What have I achieved over the past 12 weeks that I did not expect?

- What is my reward for completing 12 weeks of challenging training?

- Do I have any new goals that I would like to fulfill over the next three to six months?

You have completed twelve weeks of workouts and fitness challenges and created a great foundation, so what can you do next to keep you motivated on your fitness journey?

You can repeat this twelve week program and augment your intensity by increasing your sets, repetitions, and/or adding resistance. Another option is to purchase the Worthy Workouts book and website subscription which consists of over 100 unique circuit training routines and videos to help you reach optimal fitness throughout the year without ever doing the same routine twice. Visit **www.worthyfitness.com**.

Remember to stay connected to us through our social media community for fitness and hair tips, exercises of the week, various fitness challenges and support!

"Take care of your body. It's the only place you have to live."
— Entrepreneur, author, motivational speaker- Jim Rohn

CONGRATULATIONS!

If you've made it this far, you are ready to commit to ending the love affair with your hair. This affair has lasted far too long, and it's time for you to respect yourself enough to end it. By now, you have begun to evaluate the foods you have been eating and feeding your family. We trust you have also determined the workout schedule that works best for you. Now, we must work together to ensure you remain motivated!

The best way for you to maintain your enthusiasm is to remain connected to a community dedicated to positive transformation; we have created that environment on our **Instagram (LoveAffair_Hair)**, **Twitter (@LoveAffair_Hair)**, and **Facebook** page **(www.Facebook.com/LoveAffairWithMyHair)**. We are present online to provide encouragement, feedback, and answer your questions. You will also have the opportunity to connect with other women WORLDWIDE who are fighting a similar battle. This is a rare opportunity for you to receive direct feedback and support from the authors of this book, two fitness professionals who know your struggle, firsthand. We want nothing more than to be a partner in your successes, so please allow us the opportunity to help you through the use of our social media.

If you haven't already, use **#loveaffairwithmyhair** to profess what your hair means to you. Acknowledge your struggles so you can make a change. Please share your SMART goals with us by using **#hookupwithmyhealth**.

We are here for you! It is not uncommon to have questions when starting something new. You can ensure your questions are answered by one of us by using **#askHeather** or **#askDesiree**. Don't be shy; we are all on one team striving for one common goal!

We are so proud of you! The struggle many women of color have with their weight is deeply rooted in our history, culture, and society. Therefore, making a change goes against much of what we have been taught our entire lives. Although this journey will not always be easy, be inspired in knowing that you are helping to improve not only your health but also the health of your family and community for generations to come!

ACKNOWLEDGMENTS

Hard work goes into the creation of any book and we are fortunate enough to have had some great supporters along the way:

God, without whom none of our successes would be possible.

Together, we would like to thank our talented photographers:
Marco Antonio Iraola of Fotos by Marco in Virginia Beach, Virginia, who photographed the back covers as well as the author biographies. (www.fotosbymarco.com).

Tosin Fagbemi of Toast 2 Photography in Washington, D.C., who photographed us performing the recommended exercises in the interior of the book (www. Toast2photography.com).

We would also like to thank the wonderful ladies that made sure we looked our best during our cover shoot:
Khadine Ellis of SOHO Lashes in Chesapeake, Virginia, who gave us a glowing, natural make-up look (www.SOHOlashes.com).

Michelle Williams of Versus Salon in Virginia Beach, Virginia, who made sure our hair looked fabulous in every shot (www.versussalon.com).

We sought out the expertise of some other talented hairstylists to ensure we provided professional hair care tips and advice, including:
Fran Gray of Studio Seven Hair Salon in Irvington, NJ
Lynn Miles of Makeovers: The Beauty Beat in Summit, NJ

Graphic designers including:
Gosia Smerdel for our interior book design (photojourneynow.blogspot.com).
Keilan Roberson in Dallas, TX for our cover design (keilanroberson.com).

We cannot thank **Pam Halpin, Janet Williams, and Herman Veal** enough for their long hours spent on the editing process of this book.

INDIVIDUALLY, HEATHER WOULD LIKE TO THANK:

My parents, **Oscar and Althea Worthy,** for all of their love,
support and sacrifice since the day I was born.

My supportive best friends who love me and will always tell me the truth:
Amber Vincent, Marlynn Wheeler-Love, Jennifer Lister, Darria King and Andrea Jasmin.

My **YMCA family,** especially in Summit, NJ, and across the country
who support me in all of my endeavors.

My **athletic training family** who helped me start on the road to
success and supports me in all I do.

INDIVIDUALLY, DESIRÉE WOULD LIKE TO THANK:

My parents, **Ray and Janet Williams,** who I know love me unconditionally.

My **Hampton University family** who supports me in all I do.

My **Miss America, National Sweetheart, and Miss Virginia sisters and family**
who inspire me daily to strive for the dreams many say are unachievable.

DEDICATION

Heather would like to dedicate this book to her deceased grandparents:
Harry and Edith Clark and Oscar and Margaret Worthy.

Desirée would like to dedicate this book to her deceased grandmothers:
Mary Ella Williams and Willetta Lovejoy.

Together, Heather and Desirée would like to dedicate this book to the **black women**
who have lost their battle with chronic disease due to obesity.

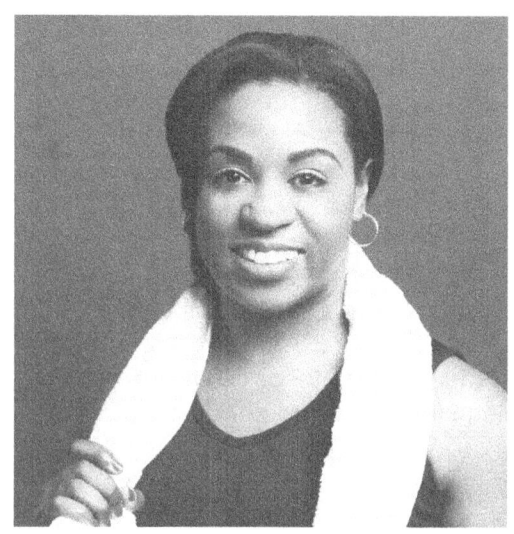

HEATHER A. WORTHY,
MSED, ATC, LAT, CPT, PES, CES

Heather Worthy, a native of Pittsburgh, PA, received her Bachelor of Science degree in Athletic Training from the University of Pittsburgh in 2002 and her Master's of Science and Education degree in Athletic Training from Old Dominion University in 2004.

From 2004 to 2005, she was the Associate Head Athletic Trainer for football and men's basketball at Hampton University. From 2005 to 2011, she served as Head Athletic Trainer for Seton Hall University's men's basketball team. She was the first, and remains the only, African American woman to work as an athletic trainer for a men's basketball program in the Big East or any other major Division I conference. She was also the Certified Athletic Trainer Minority Representative for the entire state of New Jersey.

Heather was an adjunct faculty professor for ten years and specialized in teaching Cadaver Anatomy and Therapeutic Modalities in the athletic training, physical therapy, and physician assistant graduate programs at Seton Hall University.

Heather's expertise in athletic training and health and wellness has made her a highly sought after speaker at events around the country. She was a featured speaker at the Emerging Multicultural Leadership Experience for the YMCA of the USA, African American Chamber of Commerce of Western Pennsylvania, the Big East Sports Medicine Conference, Collegiate Athletic Trainers' Society, National Athletic Trainers' Association and the Black Coaches and Administrators' Association.

Heather's muscle energy techniques and static stretching research was published in the National Journal of Athletic Training. She is a Certified and Licensed Athletic Trainer, Certified Personal Trainer, Corrective Exercise Specialist, Performance Enhancement Specialist and a Group Exercise Instructor. She has been featured in NJ Health and Beauty Magazine, NJN News, and was the personal trainer for Big Fat Mountain, a documentary about a plus sized woman's quest to climb Mt. Kilimanjaro.

She is the author of "Worthy Workouts" which was filmed, in part, as a fitness show and debuted on New Jersey's TV 36 in May 2012. Worthy Workouts was published in 2011 and serves clients and fitness professionals across the country and internationally. It was designed from an athletic standpoint with routines mimicking real life and sports movements. It is a progressive system utilizing a series of two unique circuit training routines a week for an entire year. It's the go-to-guide for personal trainers to train their clients at any fitness level. The routines are also for the intermediate to advanced exerciser who accepts the challenge to achieve a higher level of fitness.

Before becoming Regional Director of Wellness Innovation for the YMCA of Metropolitan Washington, Heather was the Wellness Director at the Summit Area YMCA in Summit, NJ. She taught her Worthy Workouts fitness class, based on the Worthy Workouts training regimen. She also created Hot Yoga Inspired Boot Camp, which integrated power yoga with strength training using weighted cork blocks. She owned a personal training company based out of NJ, Worthy Fitness, LLC, with options for studio, in-home or online training for all ages and fitness levels utilizing the book and an interactive website (www.worthyfitness.com). She specializes in individualized and small group personal training as well as sports performance training for collegiate and professional athletes, rehabilitation for active individuals and ACL prevention trainings for female athletes.

Heather lives and breathes fitness everyday and finds happiness and joy in healthy living. Whether she is teaching a fitness class, training a client, or building wellness programs, she connects with people on a deeper level and strives to develop the entire person, not just one part of them. She sees the fitness potential in everyone and meets people where they are in their lives.

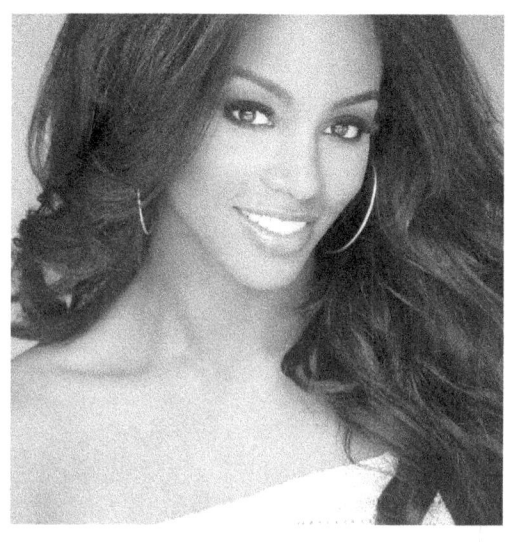

DR. DESIRÉE J. WILLIAMS,
PT, DPT, RYT-200
MISS VIRGINIA USA 2016
MISS VIRGINIA 2013

Dr. Williams is a physical therapist and an Assistant Professor in the Department of Physical Therapy at her alma mater, Hampton University. Desirée received her Doctor of Physical Therapy degree from Hampton University, where she also earned a Bachelor of Science degree in Health and Physical Education, minoring in Leadership studies. In addition to being a licensed physical therapist, Desiree is also certified to teach K-12 Health and Physical Education. Furthermore, Desirée has been a certified yoga instructor since 2009, a Reiki practitioner since 2011, and traveled to the Yunnan Province of China for seven weeks to study Community Health & Traditional Chinese Medicine.

Desirée was crowned Miss Virginia USA 2016, providing her the opportunity to compete in the 2016 Miss USA Competition. Moreover, Desiree took a yearlong sabbatical during the 2013-2014 academic year to serve as Miss Virginia 2013 and compete in the Miss America Competition. Desiree is the first African American woman to hold both state titles, and one of three women in Virginia history to hold both titles. Desirée's commitment to fitness has won her numerous Lifestyle & Fitness swimsuit awards.

Over the years, Desirée has spoken to several thousands of children and adults promoting optimal movement throughout the lifespan as well as her personal platform, Fighting Childhood Obesity: Let's Move! Desirée believes a community approach is necessary to combat the obesity epidemic.

She has also been given the opportunity to speak at dozens of schools and serve as a guest speaker for several conferences, including the Virginia NAACP State Convention and the Virginia Association for Health, Physical Education, Recreation, and Dance State Convention.

Desirée wore her hair chemically relaxed for nearly a decade before making the switch to a natural mane. Desirée now alternates between wearing her hair heat-straightened and naturally curly with plenty of workouts in between. She is excited to share her passion for health and fitness on a more global scale by writing this book and creating an online community which encourages black women and supports them through their journey.

www.ingramcontent.com/pod-product-compliance
Lightning Source LLC
Chambersburg PA
CBHW081148280526
45787CB00008B/3256

* 9 7 8 1 5 0 5 5 7 5 9 1 0 *